BIRTH-TECH
TESTS AND TECHNOLOGY IN PREGNANCY AND BIRTH

Anne Charlish
and
Linda Hughey Holt, M.D.

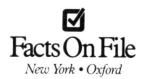

Facts On File
New York • Oxford

BIRTH-TECH

Facts On File, Inc.
460 Park Avenue South
New York NY 10016

Library of Congress Cataloging-in-Publication Data
Charlish, Anne.
  Birth-tech: tests and technology in pregnancy and birth/Anne Charlish and Linda Hughey Holt.
  p. cm.
  Includes bibliographical references.
  ISBN 0-8160-2326-3
  1. Pregnancy. 2. Prenatal diagnosis. 3. Childbirth. I. Holt, Linda Hughey. II. Title.
  RG525.C58 1990
  618.2—dc20 90-3119
                    CIP

Facts On File books are available at special discounts when purchased in bulk quantities for businesses, associations, institutions or sales promotion. Please contact the Special Sales Department of our New York office at 212/683-2244 (dial 800/322-8755 except in NY, AK or HI).

Text design by Donna Sinisgalli
Jacket design by Catherine Hyman
Composition by Facts on File, Inc.
Manufactured by Maple-Vail Manufacturing Group
Printed in the United States of America

10 9 8 7 6 5 4 3 2 1

This book is printed on acid-free paper.

Contents

Author's Note

I should like to acknowledge a great debt of gratitude to Dr. Patricia Roberts for her unfailing patience and sound advice, and to her son, Thomas, who endured maternal deprivation in the gestation of this book.

Professor Gedis Grudzinskas of the Joint Academic Unit of Obstetrics, Gynaecology and Reproductive Physiology, the London Hospital Medical College and St. Bartholomew's Hospital Medical College, London, has been most helpful, with invaluable comments. I am indebted to him for his commitment to this book.

Dr. Linda Hughey Holt, department chairman of Obstetrics and Gynecology at Rush North Shore Hospital is best known to American readers for her books, *Every Woman's Guide to Feeling Good* and *The A-Z of Women's Sexuality*. I am indebted to her, too, for her painstaking work on this edition.

Anne Charlish

Introduction

It is the hope of every prospective mother that she will be safely delivered of a normal and healthy child. Indeed, it is the expectation of most women in the Western world that this will be so. This expectation is in stark contrast to that of their mothers and grandmothers who were well aware of the risks of pregnancy and labor and that of women in many third world countries where medical research and technology still fall greatly short of the needs.

Prior to 1935, when the first antibiotic was developed, 1 in 200 to 250 pregnancies resulted in the death of the mother, most commonly from infection. Blood transfusion, more sophisticated anesthesia and the wider use of sterile techniques caused the maternal death rate to drop in 1 in 4,000 by the mid-sixties and to 1 in over 11,000 by 1987. Today the commonest cause of maternal death is hypertensive disease (raised blood pressure) and its major complication, eclampsia.

Infant deaths, which before World War II were commonly caused by infection, were by the mid-sixties, when antibiotics were freely available, mostly associated with low birth weight and congenital malformations. Diagnosis in early pregnancy and pre-pregnancy rubella immunization, together with immunization for rhesus-negative women after their first pregnancy, have reduced the number of babies born with congenital abnormalities, so that, today, the chief cause of infant death is low birth weight. Overall, the infant mortality rate has dropped from 60 per 1,000 in 1928 to 9.6 per 1,000 in 1987.

The main illnesses that may result in a low-birth-weight baby are hypertension, diabetes and severe anemia; this is why prenatal checks regularly include measurement of blood pressure, urine tests and blood tests. Regular medical investigations and assessment are essential if such diseases are to be identified and treated at an early stage.

It is increasingly recognized that the general state of the mother's health may also greatly influence the growth and development of her baby and the occurrence of complications. A woman who follows a healthy diet and avoids being overweight, and who also stops smoking and drinking alcohol before and during pregnancy, stands a better chance of producing a healthy baby of a good weight. Poor diet means poor vitamin and mineral intake and, although the fetus is able to take most of what it needs, such problems will increase with each successive pregnancy. An undetected iron deficiency may lead to anemia, which can, in turn, lead to a low-birth-weight baby.

Improvements in maternity services are geared, therefore, toward a higher standard of care for the at-risk mother, as well as for the apparently healthy mother in the lower risk category. The quality of prenatal care has to be assessed, however, from the point of view of its human relations and convenience to the patient as well as its technical efficiency. The current trend toward larger, and therefore fewer, hospital-based maternity units, away from the comforting surroundings of the family home, has introduced an impersonal and sometimes intimidating atmosphere to the process of having a baby. Efforts are constantly made to ease this situation, however, by increasing the sharing of care of the low-risk pregnant woman with her family doctor and possibly midwife in local clinics and offices.

Maternity care should be a team effort between the mother, her partner, her family doctor and the obstetric and midwifery staff who assume responsibility for her safe delivery. The important thing is communication, and some patients and doctors are better at this than others. It should be possible for prospective parents to discuss with their caregivers, in an atmosphere of mutual trust, the reasons for tests and their results, as well as the best course of action for any complications that may arise during pregnancy or labor.

Cooperation by the mother, however, is of paramount importance: A high standard of maternal care will not benefit the woman who declines to comply with the advice she receives. The mother who does not seek medical attention until her pregnancy is advanced or who fails to keep her prenatal clinic appointments will make it difficult for her midwife or obstetrician to identify a potentially serious problem in time to avert a threat to her well-being or that of her baby. Similarly, it is sensible for a mother who is an emphatic supporter of noninterference in labor and delivery to discuss her feelings fully with her midwife and/or doctor prior to the onset of labor and to retain a certain degree of flexibility in respect of her birth plan.

Many women object to a proposed induction, a Cesarean delivery or an episiotomy on the grounds that any one of these is an unnatural interference with what is considered a perfectly normal occurrence. In the case of a Cesarean delivery, some women feel remote from the delivery of their baby; but it must be stressed that this surgical procedure will probably have saved their baby's life or reduced the risk of handicap. The medical grounds for such procedures are discussed in detail in this book.

Though some people argue that there is too much technology and intervention in the natural processes of pregnancy and labor, it should be remembered that it is medical research, technology and assistance that has brought down the maternal and infant mortality rates from the unacceptably high levels of previous centuries and the early decades of this century.

Birth-Tech explains the tests and technology of pregnancy, labor and delivery in the context of how the body works in pregnancy and what happens in labor. It brings the prospective mother completely up to date with the current prenatal and delivery practices of the majority of maternity units. It also illustrates the sort of problems that the mother may encounter and, broadly, the way in which these problems may be resolved. *Birth-Tech* encourages the expectant mother to communicate with those who are looking after her and to express any doubt or anxiety, which is her right. It also emphasizes the importance of her participation in the care of herself and her unborn child.

Dr. Patricia Roberts, FRCOG
Consultant obstetrician
London, 1989

PART ONE

Weeks 0–13,
the first three months

1. Navigating the U.S. Health Care System

Birth-Tech is a book primarily about tests and procedures involved in current maternity care. It was originally written for a British audience, and American editors perusing the text could not help but be struck by the extent to which the sociology of health care delivery differed between the British and American systems. While similar tests and technology are available in both countries, the British original of *Birth-Tech* assumed that access to the tests was not an issue. In the United States, many high-tech procedures may be inaccessible to consumers due either to geographic distance or cost constraints. Before even starting to think about currently available obstetric technology, the consumer needs to have some idea of the extent to which she has access to the costlier aspects of this technology.

Most high-tech medical care in the United States is paid for either with private insurance or public funds. However, it is estimated that some 40 million Americans do not have any form of health insurance. Women of childbearing age, many of whom are young, poor and unable to work full-time due to childcare needs, are disproportionately represented among this group. While many uninsured young women are eligible for public programs offering maternity services, often such programs are themselves underfunded and may not have physicians willing to accept public-aid patients.

An uncomplicated delivery generally costs several thousand dollars for physician and hospital fees. A delivery with complications, such as a premature baby who needs intensive care, can run easily into the tens of thousands of dollars or more. Young couples need to think about these issues, preferably before conception even

3

occurs. Important issues to consider are whether you have health insurance and whether it offers maternity benefits.

Most U.S. employers offer health insurance to full-time employees. In general, part-time employees do not receive health insurance benefits. Self-employed individuals sometimes do not have health insurance and small businesses sometimes do not offer it. Furthermore, an "individual" rather than a "family" policy may not cover any pregnancy-related problems, and an increasing number of insurance policies exclude maternity coverage altogether.

If you have health insurance benefits through your job, or family coverage through your spouse's job, there are several issues that need to be investigated regarding pregnancy coverage. Was the policy valid at the time of conception? If you started a new job or acquired the insurance when you were already pregnant, some insurers will consider pregnancy a "pre-existing condition" and will refuse to cover it. Does the policy cover maternity costs for both you and the baby? There are several types of health insurance, with important distinctions. Traditional insurance, sometimes called "indemnity insurance," usually will pay a portion of medical costs after you have paid a certain initial amount called a "deductible," and a portion of the costs called a "copayment." You need to add the deductible and the copayment to estimate your total personal costs. You also have to find out how your obstetrician expects to be paid: Some doctors and midwives will bill their services directly to the insurance company, while many will expect you to pay the entire bill early in the pregnancy, leaving you to recover costs from your insurance company.

You may have the option of selecting a health maintenance organization (HMO) or a preferred provider organization (PPO) for your medical care. Typically, an HMO collects a set fee and then provides comprehensive services at little or no charge to you. However, you usually are limited to seeing their salaried physicians, and highly specialized services have to be approved. A PPO is an organization that collects insurance fees and then contracts with a panel of physicians, giving you somewhat more choice of physicians but often with greater out-of-pocket (personal) expenses than are incurred by HMO members. Indemnity insurance usually does not restrict your choice of physicians but involves larger out-of-pocket expenses.

Each of these methods of payment for health care services has its own advantages and disadvantages. If you have a choice between several different insurance plans, you can compare the physicians and benefits available. If you change plans in mid-pregnancy be sure that you do not end up losing coverage due to a pre-existing condition clause.

Unfortunately, many women find themselves already pregnant and inadequately insured. The United States is one of the few developed countries in the world that lacks some type of comprehensive publicly funded plan for maternity care, which perhaps explains why it also has one of the highest abortion rates in the world. Still, a number of programs do exist to help make maternity care available to all: If you are without adequate maternity insurance, you should, investigate local resources. Your local public health department can determine if you are eligible for public aid (Medicaid) maternity benefits and put you in touch with physicians who will accept Medicaid payments. Often hospitals operate clinics that may work on a "sliding scale" principle of matching charges to your income. Many hospitals and doctors will try very hard to set up a payment plan that is workable for families needing special fee consideration.

Fortunately, the majority of women can afford maternity care. To some extent it may depend on our priorities: When one considers that a new car may cost $10,000 or more and will be obsolete in a few years, $5,000 doesn't seem like so much for a baby! Adequate maternity care is one of the best investments we can make for the future; and we can hope that the United States will join the rest of the developed world in the next few years in making sure that maternity services are readily accessible to all.

CHOOSING A PROVIDER

American women may choose from a variety of medical-care providers for prenatal care. Your choice of provider may be dictated by availability, by insurance or financial considerations or by where you plan to have the baby. Obviously, if there is only one hospital close to you or one obstetrician or group delivering babies in your area, you will have little choice. Your insurance policy may limit your choices since it may cover only certain doctors, midwives or hospitals; if you are on public aid not all doctors and midwives will accept this form of payment. Some couples start with a place: They know where they want to deliver, and they call that hospital or birthing center for a list of individuals with delivery privileges there.

Among the providers of prenatal and delivery care you can choose from are:

1 *Obstetrician* An obstetrician is a medical doctor (M.D.) or osteopath (D.O.) who has received specialty training for four or more years in obstetrics and gynecologic surgery. Most babies in the United States are delivered by obstetricians. Most obstetricians work out of hospitals, although a few will be found in birthing centers or will offer home deliveries. Obstetricians can follow both low- and high-risk patients and perform forceps and Cesarean deliveries. "Board- certified" obstetricians have completed a rigorous written and oral exam and are recognized as specialists by the American Board of Obstetrics and Gynecology. "Board-eligible" obstetricians generally are physicians who have recently completed a residency program but have not yet taken or passed their board exams.

2 Family practitioner   A family practitioner is an M.D. or D.O. who has done specialty training in family practice, an area that includes obstetrics and office gynecology. Most family practitioners perform only low-risk obstetrics and work with an obstetrician for consultation and/or operative deliveries. Due to the high costs of malpractice insurance, many family practitioners do not currently deliver babies.

3 Perinatologist or high-risk specialist   An obstetrician who has completed additional training in high-risk obstetrics is often called a perinatologist. Most high-risk specialists or perinatologists are affiliated with large teaching hospitals, and they often treat only high-risk patients, such as severe diabetics or mothers with serious illnesses or a history of pregnancy losses.

4 Certified nurse-midwife   A nurse-midwife is a registered nurse who has completed postgraduate work in midwifery. All certified nurse-midwives (CNMs) work with a backup physician; most work in hospitals or birthing centers, and some do home deliveries. CNMs are a well-recognized part of the U.S. obstetric system.

5 Lay midwife   A person who has trained herself or who has apprenticed informally in the delivery of babies is known as a lay midwife. Since there are no standards for training and no licensure process for lay midwives, their skills vary widely. In many states lay midwifery is illegal, and lay midwives cannot obtain hospital privileges; hence they can perform home deliveries with or without any type of hospital backup.

The vast majority of American babies are born in hospitals, with a small number born at home or in freestanding birth centers. Hospitals vary, from very small medical centers that handle only normal deliveries to large tertiary-care hospitals with high- risk nurseries. Couples who are contemplating pregnancy or who are newly expectant should familiarize themselves with the options for maternity care in their area. Many hospitals and birthing centers offer guided tours or pamphlets to acquaint prospective parents with their services. There are, of course, advantages and disadvantages to any setting. A large tertiary-care center is likely to have more high-tech facilities for seriously ill mothers and babies, but may also be very busy and lacking in personalized care. A smaller unit may be quieter, but you need to make sure it has appropriate equipment and staff for unanticipated emergencies. You also need to be sure, if you have already chosen a doctor or midwife, that he or she has delivery privileges at the facility you plan to use.

Now that your financial situation has been considered and choice of physician or midwife has been made, you are ready to start the learning experience of pregnancy.

2. Your Body, Your Baby

Having a baby is for many women the most profoundly emotional and challenging experience of their entire lives. It is a time when both parents often pause to reassess their lives and to plan for the future. It is a time of great optimism, and a time, too, for doubts about one's ability not merely as a parent but as an individual.

In past centuries and the early decades of the twentieth century the joy of anticipation of having a child, and of the process of giving birth, was tempered by the knowledge that many infants died at, or shortly after, birth and that the mother's life was also at risk. The tremendous advances in medical science and technology have meant that very few women even consider such possibilities today.

We are fortunate in having at our disposal a variety of tests with which to identify for treatment any potentially dangerous conditions, such as rhesus incompatibility or undiagnosed diabetes, that can now be treated appropriately. Technological intervention has many times saved the life of a child who in previous centuries would have died. The variety of tests and technological procedures experienced by a pregnant woman these days have caused some people to question the necessity for what can seem like endless medical intervention. They may not have appreciated the medical reasons for a particular test upon a particular individual and they may also have overlooked the fact that having a baby these days is more than ten times safer for both woman and child than it was a century ago. In earlier times, when home births were the norm and medical intervention could only be minor, only the strongest individuals survived.

It is true, however, that some doctors and some hospitals may have been too quick to embrace the new technologies—induction of labor, for example—particularly in the 1970s, and this may have resulted in some women receiving more medical intervention than they required.

Some women are fearful of and others are openly hostile to doctors, whom they may regard as over-decisive, or too authoritative and "controlling." It is worth bearing in mind that doctors have to be reasonably decisive, as they are often required to make the correct decision, rapidly, in a complex situation demanding extensive medical experience. However, that is not to deny the fact that it is your body and your baby.

WHAT DO YOU NEED TO KNOW?

You have a right to know why any test is performed, how it is to be done, what the test could reveal, what the implications of any test result are and how reliable the tests have proven to be in the past. You also have an important right to know the possible outcome of a worrying test result and how you would be advised.

If, for example, you are offered a test that could identify a handicap, and if the test subsequently revealed a handicap in the fetus, you would be offered the choice of continuing the pregnancy or having an abortion. If you are opposed to abortion and know that you would not consider such a choice, then there may be no point in undergoing the test.

To give another example, some women are advised to take an amniocentesis test, although it is known that this test can cause miscarriage. Statistics, as well as your family medical history, can determine whether or not it is advisable to have the test. Consider these two cases: the statistical chance of a 20-year-old woman bearing a baby with Down's syndrome is 1 in 2,000 and her chance of miscarrying the baby through having amniocentesis is 1 in 200. It is therefore 10 times more likely that, by undergoing amniocentesis, she would miscarry the baby than bear a baby with Down's syndrome.

A 41-year-old woman, on the other hand, has the same chance of miscarrying through taking amniocentesis of 1 in 200, but her chance of bearing a Down's baby are 1 in 100. It is therefore twice as likely that she may have a handicapped baby than that the amniocentesis will cause miscarriage. The risk of having a Down's syndrome baby increases with the mother's age, at first gradually through the twenties and early thirties and then sharply from the age of 36 and each successive year until the end of the child-bearing years. At 49 years of age, for example, there is a 1 in 12 chance of a woman having a child so affected.

The crux of the matter with such tests is "consent"—specifically, whether or not you are giving an informed consent or simply agreeing to something that you do not fully understand and for which you do not have the relevant information.

Who do you ask?

If you have elected to have a home delivery, you should ask your doctor and/or midwife about anything you want to know. If you have chosen a hospital delivery, you should ask the doctor or midwife you see on a visit to the hospital. If the doctor is not available at the time you wish to inquire about a procedure, ask when you may telephone and speak to her or him.

You do not have to accept such responses as, "Oh, it's just routine," or "The doctor's busy at the moment." Follow up with "What's the aim of the routine?" or "When may I speak to her?"

Unsatisfactory answers

"We just like to keep an eye on things" is the sort of answer you may receive from a rushed doctor. You can accept that the doctor knows what he or she is doing and leave it at that, or, if you prefer, ask more specific questions and persuade the doctor to explain as fully as possible.

If you happen to be so unfortunate as to have a doctor who consistently evades questions and refuses to give you the information you seek—and this does not happen so often these days—you may want to reconsider your choice of doctors.

No news is good news

Many tests are simply routine—nothing untoward is suspected and the test is done just to be on the safe side. With such tests you may not be told the result, which to some women is quite surprising. However, if you consider the large number of routine blood tests, for example, that are carried out on hospital outpatients, it is not so surprising that you are informed only of a worrying result. However, if you wish to know the result, you may ask. It is perhaps worth asking, in any case, since this makes sure that the test result has not been mislaid and that the doctor has taken note of it.

It takes some weeks for certain test results to be known; amniocentesis results, for example, take three to four weeks, as cell cultures have to be grown. Try to establish when the result will be known and make a note for yourself to inquire at the appropriate time.

Screening tests for spina bifida involving the measurement of alphafetoprotein level (AFP test) may be repeated. There is no need to be alarmed if you are asked to have the test again. Simply remember to ask for the result of the second measurement.

Test results

In assessing the implications of any test result, you must know how reliable the test is believed to be, and you can discuss this with your doctor. You must also be aware of other factors that, taken in combination with the result of the test, could influence the eventual outcome for *you*; in other words, how healthy your baby will be. It may be difficult, for example, for a test to determine the *degree* of malfunction even if it identifies some type of handicap. Some tests, on the other hand, provide you and the doctor with a straight-forward result that needs no further interpretation.

YOUR MEDICAL RECORD

Your doctor's notes about the course of your pregnancy will be contained in your medical record. Most prenatal notes are kept on a standardized form, much of it in the form of an abbreviated "flow sheet." A copy of this record is generally sent to the hospital at which you plan to deliver. If you plan to travel or move during your pregnancy, it is a good idea to carry a copy of your prenatal record with you. Some doctors resist letting you look at or have a copy of your record, so if access to your record is an important issue to you it should be discussed early in the course of your care.

Understanding your record

To make sense of your record, not only will you need an appreciation of the tests and procedures described in later chapters, but you will also need to understand the various abbreviations used by medical staff. These include:

Ab: Abortion or miscarriage

AFP: alphafetoprotein (described in Chapter 7)

AROM: artificial rupture of membranes

BP: blood pressure

CS: Cesarean section

Ceph: cephalic

Cx: cervical smear

Ed: edema

E: engaged (baby's head)

EDC: estimated date of confinement

EDD: estimated delivery date

Eng: see E

CBC: complete blood count

FD: forceps delivery

Fe: iron

FM: fetal movement

FH: fetal heart

FHH: fetal heart heard

FMH: fetal movement heard

40T: term (the 40th and final week of pregnancy)

GTT: glucose tolerance test

H: see FHH

Hb: hemoglobin (blood count reflecting level of iron in the blood. Low Hb is the equivalent of anemia)

HBSAg: Hepatitis B surface antigen

HIV: human immuno-deficiency virus (antibodies in the blood signify a possibility of developing AIDS)

H/T: hypertension (high blood pressure)

ISCU: infant special care unit

IUD: intra-uterine contraceptive device

LB: live birth

LMP: last menstrual period

LSCS: lower segment Cesarean section or LTCS low transversec/s

Misc: miscarriage

MSU: mid-stream urine sample

NAD: nothing abnormal detected (this is sometimes abbreviated as NIL or by means of a check mark)

NTD: neural tube defect

PET: pre-eclamptic toxemia (see pre-eclampsia and toxemia)

PIH: pregnancy-induced hypertension

PP: presenting part

PT: termination of pregnancy (see Chapter 7)

SB: still birth

SFD: small for dates

SLE: systemic lupus erythematosis (a rheumatoid disease, which affects the skin, producing red blotches, and which also affects the kidneys and liver by attacking the arteries)

SRM: spontaneous rupture of membranes

STD: sexually transmitted disease

SVD: spontaneous vaginal delivery

T: see 40T

TCA: to come again

TCI to come in (to be admitted to hospital)

VDRL: venereal disease research laboratory (syphilis and gonorrhea)

VE: vaginal examination

You will also find a number of terms throughout the book. These include:

ante-partum: before delivery

cardiac: heart

cephalic: baby's head end

cephalopelvic disproportion: when the baby's head is too large for the woman's pelvis

cervical suture: stitch inserted in cervix to prevent late miscarriage or early labor. Usually inserted at 14 weeks or after.

eclampsia: convulsive stage of pre-eclampsia (see pages 36 and 42 and Chapter 5)

endocrine: of the hormone-producing glands

episiotomy: incision made in the perineum to facilitate delivery of the baby; always performed with forceps deliveries (see Chapter 11)

gestational age: age in weeks of the embryo or fetus

glycosuria: glucose in the urine

hemoglobinopathy: disease of hemoglobin formation, e.g., thalassemia, sickle cell disease

hemolytic: damaged red blood cells, causing anemia

Hb electrophoresis: test for identifying hemoglobinopathy

hydatidiform mole: a pregnancy tumor with varying degrees of malignancy (also known as molar pregnancy)

intra-partum: during labor

malpresentation: position of the baby other than the top of the head pointing directly downwards towards the mother's pelvis—e.g., breech, brow, shoulder, face

maternal abdominal length: length of the mother's abdomen

molar pregnancy: *see* hydatidiform mole, above.

neoplastic: new growth, usually cancerous

nullipara: a woman who has had no previous children

parity: number of children born to a woman, including any stillborn

percentile: a hundredth. The 50th percentile is the mean (average)

perineum: area of tissue between vagina and anus that stretches during delivery of the baby's head

placenta/placental: part of the pregnancy tissue that allows for transfer of nutrients and oxygen to the baby from the mother and removal of waste substances (including carbon dioxide) from the baby which are excreted with the mother's waste products

postpartum: after delivery

pre-eclampsia: precursor to the very serious condition of convulsions in pregnancy, known as eclampsia, which can prove fatal (described more fully in Chapter 5)

premature: baby born before 37 weeks, before which stage the lungs may have not reached complete maturity

preterm: baby born before 37 weeks

primigravida: during the first pregnancy

proteinuria: albumen (protein) in the urine

puerperium: first six weeks of the baby's life after delivery

renal: of the kidneys

rhesus factor: see Chapter 5

rubella: German measles

sickle cell or trait: see Chapter 5

thalassemia: see Chapter 5

thromboembolic: blood clots in veins, which may then be
   conducted to other parts of the body through the circulation
toxemia: term formerly used to describe a hypertensive state
   seen only in pregnancy, which, if untreated, will lead to
   convulsions in the baby and the mother. Now known as
   pre-eclampsia
uterine anomaly: congenital malformation of the uterus
vertex: top of head

As your pregnancy continues, many of these terms fall into place,
and you may surprise yourself at your grasp of medical terminol-
ogy by the time your pregnancy "comes to term" (you are ready to
deliver). Reading and understanding your medical record may
help you feel more in control of your body, your pregnancy,
medical procedures and, eventually, your admission to the hospital for the birth. You may feel happier, however, to leave everything to the medical and nursing staff and simply let them get on
with it—many women do! Whether or not you understand the
details of what is going on is not likely to affect the *outcome* of your
pregnancy, merely, perhaps, how you *feel* about it.

Preparation for pregnancy, both mentally and physically, is an
important factor in how you will feel during the pregnancy and
how you will respond to your new baby. There is much you can
do to help yourself prepare for pregnancy and this is the subject of
the next chapter.

3. The Best of Health

Taking care of yourself before and during pregnancy is important for the healthy development of the fetus so that your child has the best possible start in life. You will also be able to withstand fatigue, cope with the process of birth better, recover more rapidly, and prepare yourself for the challenges of parenthood, the first months of which are inevitably tiring for most women. Enough rest, a well-balanced healthful diet, and regular exercise are vital to your developing pregnancy. This would be a good time to quit smoking, and limit alcohol intake to two or three glasses of wine a week at most.

Many women feel exceptionally healthy during pregnancy, particularly in the middle three months, when their hair and skin takes on a glow of vitality. For others, however, nausea, constant fatigue and all sorts of minor aches and pains dominate. If you are already pregnant, there is much you can do to help yourself.

SLEEP

Everyone needs a different amount of sleep each night. Only you can tell if you are not getting enough. The important thing is not to let yourself become too tired to cope. The *timing* of the sleep you get is just as important as the *amount*. You will benefit most by going to bed at roughly the same time each evening and getting up at the same time the following morning: In this way your sleep patterns become regularized. If you go to bed very late, you will probably find that you cannot recoup the sleep you need by sleeping in the following morning, and you will feel tired all day.

Remember to avoid lying or sleeping on your back too much; this may feel comfortable but it does impede your circulation and can therefore lead to insufficient oxygen reaching your baby, to you feeling cold and your ankles and wrists swelling.

As you approach the last three months of pregnancy, you may find that you need more sleep than before. Try going to bed an hour or two earlier than usual and you may feel better within a week. Even if you don't sleep straight away, just resting quietly will benefit you and your growing baby. Taking an afternoon rest is a great luxury that often benefits expectant mothers, but if you are working you will of course be able to do this only on weekends. As your pregnancy advances, you will probably find it helpful to leave work an hour earlier, if you can, so that you travel out of the rush hour and arrive home knowing that you can have a hour's rest without disrupting the evening's normal schedule.

If you already have one child or more, encourage your partner to look after them as much as possible—from getting the supper and playing games to helping with homework and bath time. After all, he will have to know how to do all this when the new baby arrives.

DIET

Everyone must by now be aware that a pregnant woman does not need to "eat for two." This will result not so much in a healthy, bouncing baby but in an excessively overweight mother who feels worn out merely by walking up the stairs and whose clothes don't fit her! All you need to remember is to eat from the four main food groups (see below) each day and to eat three times a day or more, with the lightest meal taken in the evening. For optimum health, cut out coffee, alcohol, sugar, cakes, sweets and highly processed foods containing a lot of additives and preservatives. You should avoid products that contain unpasteurized milk, lightly cooked or raw eggs (see page 18), and rare or raw meats.

1. protein in the form of meat, fish, eggs
2. smaller amounts of protein and calcium from dairy products such as cheese, milk and milk products
3. "second class" proteins from nuts, peas, beans, lentils and soy beans. Peas and beans, as well as other vegetables, provide you with essential vitamins. Spinach is particularly useful in pregnancy, as are most of the fruits, especially oranges and apples.
4. fiber from seeds and grains (and to a much lesser extent from fruit and vegetables) in the form of barley and bran, for example. Eat one of the following at least once a day: wholewheat cereal, wholewheat bread, wholegrain pasta.

Try to make your diet as varied as possible. If you have some extra milk, cheese and yogurt, you should not experience the calcium deficiency that sometimes occurs in pregnancy. (The growing baby needs substantial amounts of calcium for the healthy development of its bones.) Milk and cheese are excellent forms of calcium and protein. Add grated cheese to salads and to pasta dishes. If you normally drink coffee and tea through the day, substitute these drinks alternately with milk and pure fruit juices. Milk provides you and the baby with extra calcium and the fruit juices with essential vitamins.

Coffee, and tea, too, to some extent, are essentially drugs that stimulate the action of the heart and the digestive system. This can cause feelings of anxiety and because of the quick lift that both drinks provide they disguise fatigue. It would be better not to have the coffee, to feel tired and take a rest, or go to bed earlier. All cola drinks contain caffeine and they should be eliminated from the diet completely. They have no beneficial effect and the gases that they contain tend to cause bloating.

Many pregnant women suffer from constipation during their pregnancies, but this can be avoided by eating lots of foods containing fiber—such as wholegrain cereals, wholegrain bread and wholegrain spaghetti and other pasta. If you find that you are still constipated, add 1 tablespoon of 40-percent bran to your cereal or fruit salad, but no more than one a day.

Iron deficiency is quite common in pregnancy, but this too can be avoided by eating iron-rich foods such as liver and kidneys, fish, eggs and leafy green vegetables, spinach in particular. Eating these foods will also provide you with the zinc that you need. If you eat regularly from the four main food groups, you should not need to buy any vitamin or mineral supplements. Nonetheless, most doctors recommend prenatal vitamins to be certain you are getting the essential nutrients. If you become anemic during pregnancy, you will be given iron (Fe). There is no benefit to be gained by taking too much iron as any surplus is excreted out of the system. Iron tablets also contribute to constipation.

Preparing your food
Of almost equal importance to what foods you eat is their method of preparation. For example, if you eat four-day-old vegetables boiled until they are soft, you will have reduced considerably their vitamin content, to the extent that it would have been more beneficial to have eaten frozen peas.

Meat The main principle that meat-eaters need to remember is to cut down on fat. Baking, broiling and microwaving are the best methods of cooking, using the least amount of fat in which to cook the meat. When you switch from frying to broiling, you may be surprised at the amount of fat that the meat itself contains: you certainly do not need to add any! Cut off any excess fat and do not eat skin—chicken skin, for example—which is fatty.

Fat is the most fattening food that exists, which is one good reason for avoiding it. A second is that it can lead to heart disease; a third is that it has little nutritional value; and a fourth is that it can lead to constipation. Of all foods, fats stay in the stomach longest and they therefore slow down your digestive processes. Fat is a source of vitamins, however, and also provides energy, particularly in cold weather.

Fish   Again, try to avoid excess fat. Plain white fish such as sole or flounder are healthier than fatty fish, such as mackerel and herring. If you have a microwave, use it to cook fish, as it retains the moisture and flavor better than any other method. Avoid frying, as that would mean adding fat or oil to the fish. Grilling or poaching are healthy alternatives to microwaving.

Eggs   In Great Britain in 1988, salmonella, a dangerous bacterial infection, was found in eggs. In the United States, eggs are probably safe, but should not be eaten raw. Pregnant women are advised to avoid homemade mayonnaise, Caesar salad, soft-cooked eggs (such as poached, soft-boiled and fried with runny yolks), and other raw or lightly cooked egg preparations.

Vegetables   A lot of the goodness, in the form of vitamins, is lost when you boil vegetables, so cook them for the minimum possible time. Alternatively, steam them or microwave them. Try to eat as many different vegetables as you can and as often as possible, so that you eat them at peak freshness. Raw, fresh vegetables are best of all: try not only tomatoes, cucumber, radishes, lettuce and onion but also Chinese cabbage, spinach, kale, chopped white cabbage, mushrooms, broccoli, cauliflower, grated carrot—all taste even better in their raw state. Prepare them as close as possible to your meal time as their vitamin content decreases after prolonged exposure to air.

It does not matter whether you are already some weeks into your pregnancy or not: following a good and varied diet will benefit both you and your baby provided that you start right away. The ideal is to be as healthy as possible before you conceive; if you are not, it is still worth starting a healthy life-style at four months or even five months into your pregnancy.

EXERCISE AND FRESH AIR

One of the most important aspects of exercising daily for a pregnant woman is the exposure to fresh air and sunlight. Performing exercises in the privacy of your bedroom is good for you, but you can double the benefit by doing the same exercises outdoors on a sunny day or by taking a good, long walk each day. Sunlight is essential for the formation of vitamin D and your lungs benefit by breathing in fresh air rather than the stale air of your workplace or your home.

Sports to be avoided during pregnancy include squash, riding, skiing, water skiing, windsurfing and any that you know could cause you awkward, sudden movements or a heavy fall. Swimming is without doubt the best exercise for the pregnant woman. You are weightless in the water and you can therefore increase your suppleness and stamina, without the sensation of making an effort. Provided that you swim in a public pool with an attendant, the risks are few—choose one that you know is well run and frequently cleaned out. Unlike every other sport, you can continue swimming until you are in an advanced stage of pregnancy; and you can do it at any time of the year, with or without a friend.

Walking, in flat shoes that provide support, is also good for you, but it will not increase your level of fitness unless you walk each day for about 15 minutes at a brisk pace.

The purpose of exercise, in principle, is to increase stamina, suppleness and strength. Some forms of exercise, such as swimming, can help with all three, while others, such as tennis, deal with only one of the three requirements. Exercise also tones up the muscles, which will be of great benefit to you in the process of giving birth, and revitalizes the cardiovascular system. The heart muscle is the center of this system and its efficient functioning is therefore vital: Exercise helps to tone the muscle, causing blood to be pumped more efficiently around the body. This ensures that freshly oxygenated blood reaches the tissues more rapidly and that waste products are excreted more quickly and regularly, thus helping to prevent feelings of sluggishness and constipation, and preventing the various characteristic aches and pains of pregnancy.

You may wish to carry out a daily routine of exercises as well as some form of outdoor exercise. Certain exercises are designed to increase either suppleness, strength or stamina, or a combination of any of these three. Suppleness, particularly of the pelvic muscles, may do much to help you through the pain of birth. Breathing exercises are also valuable; you can learn about these from prenatal or childbirth preparation classes. (Contact American Society for Psychoprophylaxis in Obstetrics, Inc. [ASPO/Lamaze] for information or ask your doctor for details if you have not already been told and see also Chapter 8.)

Before you embark on any form of exercise or a program of exercises, check with your doctor that it is safe to do so. Do not do anything that you know you would have found strenuous even before you were pregnant. If you experience any of the following, stop exercising immediately and rest; if any of the symptoms persist for more than 5–10 minutes, consult your doctor:

1. breathlessness
2. dizziness
3. pain or feeling of tightness in the abdominal area, chest, arms, back or joints
4. any sort of headache
5. unusual fatigue or feeling of inertia
6. cramping in your lower abdomen
7. vaginal bleeding

It is essential not to overdo things during your pregnancy: Your body is already working hard every minute of the day as it copes with the demands of the baby growing inside you, so do not ask too much of your body. The ideal is fitness, not frenzy and fatigue, which could present risks for both you and the baby.

Exercises
Ten to 15 minutes a day of a varied program of exercises is sufficient to keep you in shape. Choose from the following, but do not devote an entire session to any one particular exercise. Each exercise is designed to achieve one or more of the different types of fitness that you need in pregnancy and giving birth: deep even breathing; improved muscle tone, particularly in the muscles of the back and the pelvis; relaxation; good posture, in order to avoid the backache typical of pregnancy; good circulation in order to make sure that both you and the baby receive sufficient oxygen and to prevent swelling at your wrists and ankles.

1 Controlling your breathing   Breathlessness is a common occurrence in pregnancy, but you can overcome this to some extent by learning to control your breathing. Some women find it easier to manage labor and birth by remembering their breathing exercises, and breathing in accordance with contractions.
Place a pillow on the floor to support your head, and lie down. Make a conscious effort to relax, breathing moderately and slowly to avoid dizziness. Place your hands on either side of your body, where you can feel your lower ribs, and breathe in and out, feeling your body rise and fall as you breathe first in, then out. When you breathe in, breathe in through your nose, and then breathe out through your mouth, blowing lightly at the same time.
Continue with this moderate and slow breathing exercise, which is also, incidentally, a wonderful method of relaxation. As you breathe in, feel your abdominal area rise; as you breathe out, contract your abdominal muscles and force the air out of your mouth.
When you are giving birth, regular even breathing helps to ensure that both you and the baby receive sufficient oxygen. It can also help to take the edge off the pain. During labor you will need

to push as you breathe out, but this should not be practiced during pregnancy. Just before you are about to deliver, you will be asked not to push, despite an overwhelming urge to do exactly that, while either midwife or doctor checks that the umbilical cord is safely positioned for the baby to be born. The way to do this is to breathe out or blow softly or pant, and this is something you can practice during pregnancy. It is very important for you not to push when you are instructed not to in case the baby is expelled too forcibly, incurring severe tears of the perineum.

2 Back exercises Even if your back aches badly, do not arch backwards in an attempt to relieve it and, if you are doing exercises on all fours, do not let your back dip. The best method of quick relief is to lean forwards from the waist for a minute or two, or to lie down on your side with your back in a curve.

Any back exercises that you may have learned before you became pregnant should be carried out with care and only with the advance approval of your doctor. Some back exercises are quite strenuous and are not recommended for pregnant women.

Bending and stretching exercises help to increase suppleness in your back muscles, thus enabling them to bear the increased weight of your body more easily and with less likelihood of strain.

Lie down on the floor with a pillow for your head. Have your arms out flat a little distance from your body with the palms of your hands facing up. Extend your legs fully by stretching your toes away from you and then bringing them towards you. You should be able to feel the back of your legs and your back pressing against the floor. In order to get the upper part of your back fully relaxed against the floor, first pull your shoulder blades together and then relax them, breathing out deeply at the same time. These movements not only help to strengthen the muscles of your back and calves but also encourage you to relax.

Next bend your knees up, keeping your back as close to the floor as possible. Bring your head forward so that it is half-way to making a right angle with your chest, and breathe in slowly. Now breathe out, raising the upper part of your body but keeping your waist upon the floor. Return slowly to a lying position and make a conscious effort to relax.

Provided that you feel sufficiently fit, and you are experiencing none of the warning signs listed on page 20, you can progress to holding out your arms in front of you while performing the same exercise and, after a few weeks, to clasping your hands behind your head. You will find that these progressions make your exercise sessions just a little more strenuous; provided that you are in shape, this should not present a problem. Remember, though, that all exercising and exercises must be carried out regularly and systematically: progression is the keynote. Not only will it prove counterproductive, but it could also be hazardous, both for you and the baby, if you launch yourself into a frenzied exercise session from a starting point of complete unfitness. If in doubt, check with your doctor or consultant.

3   Pelvis and pelvic floor exercises   These exercises are designed principally to loosen up your pelvic muscles, which will be of great value to you when you give birth and will also help you to return to shape after the birth; they also help to develop your back muscles and encourage you to moderate your breathing.

Get down on the floor on all fours and then arch your back a little upwards. Now let it return to the normal all-fours position—but do not let it dip. As you do this exercise, you should be able to feel your pelvis move up and down. Now move your pelvis from side to side like a dog wagging its tail: You may feel silly, but the benefit of supple, strong pelvic muscles cannot be overemphasized. Repeat these exercises several times.

Now stand up with your feet a little apart and your legs slightly bent at the knee. Move your pelvis first to one side and then to the other, and then from front to back, and back again. As you perform these movements, concentrate on contracting and relaxing the muscles of the vagina and anus: Imagine that you are urinating, then forcibly stopping yourself and starting again. Here you are exercising those muscles that are likely to be stretched to their utmost during the birth; if they are accustomed to stretching and contracting, it is more likely that they will regain their elasticity after the birth. Good muscular control in this area also helps to prevent the involuntary urination (incontinence) common during pregnancy and the months after the birth.

A variation on what is known as the pelvic tilt is to stand against a wall with your head, back and bottom touching the wall. Your feet are a little away from the wall and a short distance apart. Bend slightly at the knees to increase the contact of your head, back and bottom to the wall. Push the lower part of your back against the wall, tightening your stomach muscles at the same time and tilting your pelvis forward and up. Your shoulders should remain against the wall as you count to 3—and now relax, allowing your bottom to make contact with the wall. Repeat the exercise several times. You will find with practice that you can synchronize your breathing so that you breathe in and out rhythmically as you contract and relax your muscles. This exercise also develops and strengthens the muscles of your lower back so that you are less likely to suffer from backache.

Privacy is not required for most of these exercises, so you can do them in the evening watching television or at lunchtime, if you work. The best time of all for any exercise is the morning, if you are prepared to get up 15 minutes earlier than usual.

4 *Circulation* Clearly, the best exercise to keep your circulation moving and to make sure that the baby receives enough freshly oxygenated blood is to keep moving around, but you also need rest and so does the baby. Remember to avoid lying for long periods on your back; lie instead on your side. Wrist and ankle exercises are effective in keeping the circulation moving, even when you are compelled to be sedentary, such as when traveling, eating, watching television, waiting to be seen at the doctor's office or reading. Flex your fingers and move your wrists around in a circle and then back again in the opposite direction. Do this with both hands several times. Make the same movements with your feet, preferably with shoes removed. Wriggle your toes vigorously and stretch your ankles from side to side and around in a circle and back again.

Make a note of how much time you are devoting to exercising and try to increase it by five minutes or so every 2 to 3 weeks. Do not be tempted to overdo things, for the reasons stated earlier. The time spent in regular, methodical exercise will repay you with good dividends and, in the short term, is a marvelous way of relaxing.

NO SMOKING

Giving up smoking is the single most important thing you can do to help yourself in pregnancy and to give your growing child a healthy start in life.

Even if you were not to get enough sleep, never exercised and did not eat particularly wisely, the fact that you continued to smoke in the first few months of your baby's life—while you are carrying her or him—is still the most potentially harmful influence on your child's health. Women who smoke during pregnancy are more likely to miscarry or to have a stillbirth; if they carry the baby to term the baby is likely to be underweight (usually referred to as low birth weight); and the child is more likely to suffer with infections of the respiratory tract, such as bronchitis and colds. The child's ability to concentrate and learn may also be affected, as may his or her capacity for memory. Babies of low birth weight are dysmature: Although they are of the correct age to be delivered, they will not be as fully developed as the baby of normal weight and will therefore be more vulnerable to infection and disease.

If you are already pregnant and still smoking, don't be tempted to think "Well, it's too late now." It is not. You can minimize the damage by giving up now, or, if you cannot, by cutting down drastically with the aim of giving up in two weeks.

Nicotine is a drug which, like many others, is addictive, and it is therefore undeniably difficult to kick the habit. While you are doing so, remember two things: firstly, if you give it up now, you'll never have to suffer the withdrawal symptoms again; secondly, you are doing your best to make sure that you give birth to a healthy and active child. Remind yourself, too, that not only are you storing trouble for your child if you continue to smoke but also for yourself as well. If you have a child who suffers continually with bronchitis and who also finds it difficult to concentrate, you will be mother to a child who is out of school more frequently than her or his classmates and who makes slower progress in school than the others because of the inability to concentrate. In the early years before school your child will be difficult to keep amused and you may hear yourself exclaiming to other mothers, or the doctor, "He can't seem to concentrate on anything for more than two minutes."

Nicotine is a dangerous drug that kills some 380,000 people in the U.S. alone each year. Women who smoke are twice as likely as nonsmokers to develop cervical cancer. So give up smoking. First of all, set the scene. Get rid of ashtrays, lighters, cigarettes and matches. If your partner smokes, establish with him the day that you are both to give up. (Not only is it exceedingly difficult to give up smoking when there is a smoker in the house, but also you and your child are still exposed to some of the injurious effects of smoking if you inhabit a smoky atmosphere. This is known as "passive smoking.")

Right away, declare some of the rooms of your home as no-smoking zones: Go for the bedroom and bathroom first, perhaps, followed by the kitchen, leaving the living room until last.

Make a conscious effort not to light up in the morning and hold out as long as you can. Research has shown that the later you start to smoke in the day, the lower the number of cigarettes per hour that you will smoke. It is not simply that you smoke fewer because you started later in the day: the rate at which you smoke is also correspondingly lower. Push your starting time further and further back, until you are smoking only one or two in the evening and those in the living room, the other areas of the house having been declared no-smoking zones.

If you weaken, or catch a whiff of someone else's cigarette, concentrate on the truly foul smell of an old ashtray or a smoky bus, and compare it with the delightful smell of a newborn baby—a pure, sweet smell like no other. Try to remember, too, that nicotine goes directly into your bloodstream—and therefore directly into your baby's as well.

Giving up smoking sometimes causes weight gain, partly because people tend to nibble instead of smoke and partly also because, in the absence of nicotine, the metabolism can slow a little and thus less energy is used up and more food converted to fat. Don't let this worry you too much at this stage (your doctor will tell you if you are putting on much too much weight), for you should be able to shed most of it after the birth through breast feeding and having lots more to do.

Lastly, do your best to avoid smoky atmospheres—since this can prove harmful to you and the baby, too—such as bars, parties, and the homes of friends who you know will not refrain from smoking.

ALCOHOL

It is now known that the sperm of men who are heavy drinkers can produce babies with serious defects and that women who drink, either around the time of conception or during pregnancy, can give birth to severely damaged babies. Some doctors maintain that an occasional drink will do no harm, while others advocate giving it up altogether. All are agreed that heavy, regular drinking or drinking in binges can carry very high risks for the baby and can cause abnormality.

An occasional glass of wine may do no harm; any more than that should be regarded as too much. Hard liquor contains much more alcohol than wine or beer and should be avoided completely during pregnancy.

If you have already had one child with a severe abnormality, your partner should consider giving up drinking for three months before conception and until after you are sure that you are pregnant, and you should refrain from drinking throughout the pregnancy.

Babies born to heavy drinkers may be affected by alcohol in what is known as the fetal alcohol syndrome. This syndrome comprises a pattern of physical and mental defects that includes severe growth deficiency, heart defects, malformed facial features, a small head, abnormalities of coordination and movement, and mental impairment. Babies so afflicted may be born addicted to alcohol and may suffer withdrawal symptoms, so that they seem twitchy and restless. They cannot feed properly and will not thrive. They have to be sedated with drugs such as valium to help them through the withdrawal phase.

OTHER DRUGS

If you are pregnant, or likely to be so, remind your doctor of this at any time that he or she prescribes a drug for you. If you are hoping to have a baby but are not yet definitely known to be pregnant, do make sure that you remind the doctor of this *each* and *every* time you accept a prescription.

Avoid all over-the-counter drugs and check first with your doctor, however innocuous you believe the medication to be. Aspirin is to be avoided in pregnancy and some cough syrups, for example, contain substances that would be harmful to the growing baby. Ergotamine, sometimes prescribed for migraine, can lead to miscarriage. Some diuretics can cause low potassium levels. Antibiotics such as tetracycline taken during pregnancy later cause the baby's teeth to be stained yellow. Therefore, consult with your doctor and remind him or her that you are asking because you are pregnant or may be so. This applies particularly if you are seeing a different doctor from the one you normally see.

ILLEGAL DRUGS

Illegal drugs have been deemed so because they are highly dangerous unless taken under medical supervision. If you are pregnant such drugs, which include heroin, morphine, amphetamines, crack and cocaine, are highly dangerous not only to you but also to your baby. Such drugs must not be taken. All cause withdrawal symptoms in the baby if taken in the eighth to ninth months of pregnancy. There is also a danger of contracting AIDS when sharing needles to inject drugs intravenously. Crack and cocaine are particularly dangerous, since they can trigger placental separation (abruption) and loss of the baby. Treatment programs are available for pregnant women.

X-RAYS

You may have an X-ray in pregnancy but only under exceptional circumstances. If you are pregnant or hope to be so you *must* be sure to remind any medical or nursing staff of this if they propose X-raying you. You must also be sure to tell your dentist. Routine dental X-rays can nearly always wait until after the birth and it would be better to put them off. When dental X-rays are necessary you should wear a leaded abdominal shield.

The Oxford Survey, the largest ever of its kind, covers all cases of childhood cancers in England, Scotland and Wales from the years 1953 to 1979. It has identified an incidence of cancer twice as high in children of X-rayed mothers as those whose mothers were not exposed to radiation in pregnancy. It seems that human sensitivity to X-rays is very high in the first 12 weeks of pregnancy. In the past, experts have relied on the evidence that the embryos of animals do not appear to be any more sensitive to X-rays than the grown animal. It has been assumed, therefore, that the same may apply to humans. The Oxford Survey appears to turn this belief on its head and the best advice for pregnant women now must be to avoid X-rays except in cases of medical necessity.

It was said at the start of this chapter that there is much you can do to help yourself and improve your health if you are already pregnant. If you are not yet pregnant, there are a number of other matters to consider, which come under the general headings of preconceptual care and genetic counseling.

Sufficient sleep, a sensible diet, plenty of exercise and fresh air, giving up smoking, taking only an occasional drink, avoiding other drugs and refusing X-rays unless considered essential, can all be included as optimum preconceptual care. There is no doubt that you can do much to improve your own health and that of your future baby's by looking after yourself as described in the earlier pages of this chapter. It is also important that your partner cuts out or cuts down on alcohol in the preconception phase. You are less likely to become pregnant, and abnormalities are more likely to occur in the child, if your partner drinks regularly. For sperm to be at their healthiest, your partner needs to observe the advice concerning sleep, diet and giving up smoking, as well as giving up alcohol. Once you have conceived, your partner may revert to his normal lifestyle if he so wishes, with the exception of continuing not to smoke.

If you are not already pregnant, there are a number of health checks that you may undergo in order to eliminate the possibility of certain problems that would be difficult to treat if you were pregnant. These include Pap smear test, breast examination, rubella immunity test, mumps immunity test, dental check, herpes check, and AIDS testing. You should also stop taking any contraceptive pill and any other drug for some time before attempting to conceive (the length of time depends on the drug and your doctor's advice concerning how long it is thought that particular drug remains in your bloodstream).

If you suspect that you have been exposed to the risk of autoimmune deficiency syndrome (AIDS), you may consider having a blood test in order to determine whether or not you have contracted the virus. The virus can be transmitted to the fetus by the mother, and it may eventually kill you and the child. If you have AIDS or are HIV-positive, you would be wise not to become pregnant.

If you suffer from any of the following conditions, you are recommended to discuss your planned pregnancy with your obstetrician and/or a genetic counselor. No one will advise you not to have a child: they will simply tell you what the statistical risks to you and a child would be. With special medical management from the start, you may well be told that there is no reason why you may not bear a healthy, normal child. Tests can be carried out before you attempt to conceive to determine your chances, and this is an aspect of medical technology that no one should refuse, for it can provide you with the peace of mind necessary for a happy pregnancy. The conditions are epilepsy, diabetes, hypertension (high blood pressure), asthma requiring that steroids be taken, heart murmur, heart or kidney disease, a history of miscarriage, fetal abnormality or problems in previous pregnancies. A genetic counselor's advice may prove invaluable if you have been trying to become pregnant for over a year and fear that you may be infertile.

There exist a number of hereditary diseases, and if any of these is present in your family you may worry that you may bear a child so afflicted. However, it is now possible to test for many hereditary diseases at the preconceptual stage. It may be that you and your partner are free of the particular disease that you are worried about; in other words, your genes are not imprinted with the disease, and your child will not inherit it. This sort of testing is known as DNA testing and can be obtained by asking your doctor to refer you to a genetic counselor. These hereditary diseases include cystic fibrosis, Down's syndrome, Huntington's Chorea, thalassemia, sickle cell disease, Tay Sachs disease, muscular dystrophy and many other extremely rare diseases. The more common hereditary diseases are discussed in more detail in Chapter 5; see also page 157.

THE ENVIRONMENT

Having discussed what you can do yourself to improve your health, as well as what medical science has to offer, there remain a number of environmental factors to be mentioned in the context of preconceptual care. These include lead pollution, radiation from visual display terminals (VDTs) and general health and hygiene.

Lead pollution

Lead pollution, in the form of vehicle emissions, has been linked to low birth weight and impaired development of speech, memory, learning and intelligence. While living in urban areas, pregnant women may be advised to travel during non-rush hours or when pollution levels are otherwise low. Although many urban communities are making headway against leaded fuel and other automotive emissions, lead from industrial pollutants may still affect the air. Prolonged exposure to environmental pollution may have an impact on a developing fetus.

Computer terminals

Medical opinion is still divided over whether a VDT can emit sufficient radiation to injure a developing fetus. If you prefer to be cautious, avoid using them if you are pregnant or wish to be so. Alternatively, invest in a rather cumbersome lead apron to wear whenever you use such a machine.

General health and hygiene

It was reported in 1988 that children who watch excessive amounts of television are receiving certain small quantities of radiation, the effects of which are not fully understood. Also, the amount of TV watching that may become harmful is unknown. It is impossible to draw any conclusions from the tentative nature of such evidence, nor to extrapolate what may be the effect on the developing fetus of its mother watching television all day. It can only be said that watching television for more than four or five hours a day is probably as injurious to mind as to body and would therefore be better avoided.

If you have absorbed the rest of this chapter, there remain only a few matters of general hygiene to observe before and during your pregnancy. The main point of good personal hygiene is to reduce the possibility of picking up an infection that could be transmitted to the fetus or which would need to be treated with drugs that could be injurious to the growing baby. Matters such as washing one's hands after using the toilet, showering or bathing once a day, washing one's hands before handling food, discarding any food that might be "bad," and keeping cooked meats separately from raw meats in order to prevent contamination, should all be regarded as routine.

When you are pregnant avoid contact with kittens and cats and their litter and feces. Such contact can lead to infection in you (which may be mild to severe) and, more seriously, congenital birth defects in your child, in a condition known as toxoplasmosis. Contact with parrots should also be avoided for fear of the rare disease, psittacosis. Lastly, on the matter of personal hygiene, do not use so-called feminine deodorant sprays, do not douche, and avoid soaping the vaginal area more than once a day. Nonmedicated and nonperfumed soaps are recommended. If you have the occasional spotting or small show of blood, use pads in preference to tampons. (If the bleeding amounts to anything more than spotting, you should consult your doctor immediately and lie down or keep still until he or she is satisfied that nothing is amiss.)

CONFIRMATION OF YOUR PREGNANCY

Keeping yourself in the best of health is a desirable ideal both during pregnancy and to help you withstand the physical and emotional rigors of birth and the early days of parenthood. As you read this, you may already know that you are pregnant, in which case you may skip the next chapter and turn to Chapter 5. Remember that pregnancy tests taken too early can give false negative results, and, occasionally, false positive results. It is best to wait until six weeks after your last period or two weeks after a missed period before taking a pregnancy test for a higher degree of reliability unless you need to monitor earlier at your doctor's recommendation. The types of tests available and how to obtain them are described in the next chapter.

4. How do you know you're pregnant?

Some women say that they know they are pregnant from the first, before they have experienced any of the common symptoms of pregnancy. This may be natural instinct coming to the fore or it may be simply the manifestation of hoping and wishing to be pregnant. Most women do not realize that they are pregnant until they notice some of the common symptoms, and even then some women do not guess that they are pregnant until a pregnancy test provides the evidence.

The sequence of events leading to the establishment of a pregnancy is *ovulation* (the release of an egg from the woman's ovary), *fertilization* (by the man's sperm) and *implantation* of the fertilized egg, normally in the wall of the uterus. Implantation is also regarded as the moment of conception. The woman's egg is fertilized by the man's sperm, in the Fallopian tube, usually within 48 hours of the woman ovulating. Implantation, the moment of conception, then takes place, normally in the wall of the uterus, some seven days later. (See Figure 1.)

It can be difficult to pinpoint the time of conception, because periods can be very irregular, so, although it is known that implantation occurs several days after fertilization and fertilization takes place within 48 hours of the woman ovulating, it is not always possible to calculate when ovulation occurred. Ovulation takes place 14 days before the expected next period. This is not quite the same as saying it takes place 14 days after the last period, as women's menstrual cycles vary in length from 21–38 days. The 28-day cycle is the most common.

It is important to establish when implantation, or the moment of conception, took place as it is at that time that that part of the embryo (the fertilized egg) deemed to become the placenta pro-

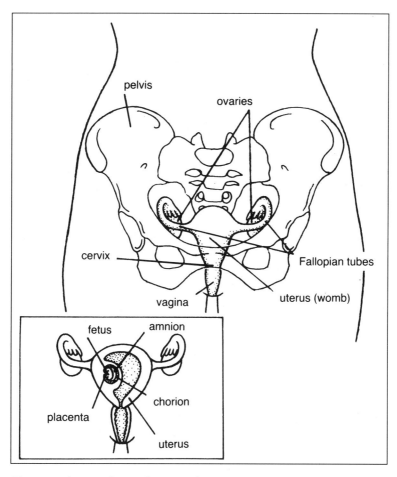

Figure 1. *A woman's sexual, or reproductive, organs comprise the uterus, the Fallopian tubes, the cervix and the vagina, and these lie within the pelvis or pelvic girdle. One of the ovaries releases an egg which is fertilized in the Fallopian tube. This travels down into the uterus where it implants, when it is known first as an embryo and later as a fetus. The inset drawing shows an embryo at about 4 weeks after implantation. At around 7–8 weeks the fetus will be enclosed by its two protective membranes, the chorion and the amnion, and it will be nourished by the placenta, which will have formed from part of the embryo.*

duces masses of a substance known as human chorionic gonadotrophin (HCG), the existence of which is crucial to early pregnancy testing.

As periods can be very irregular, it is difficult to pinpoint the time of ovulation, except by changes in the woman's body temperature or by an ovulation predictor test. This test detects the presence of luteinizing hormone (LH), which cross-reacts with HCG. Without daily temperature testing or the use of an ovulation predictor, it would be difficult to calculate the time of conception. Within seven to ten days of conception taking place, masses of HCG is produced. The presence of this substance in the woman's blood and urine is the basis of preliminary diagnosis of pregnancy. All pregnancy tests, whether carried out by your doctor, a midwife or a hospital, or by yourself using over-the-counter pregnancy testing kits, currently measure HCG. (This is discussed in more detail later in this chapter.)

COMMON SYMPTOMS OF PREGNANCY

The most common symptom of pregnancy, and the most likely event to make you visit your doctor, is a missed period. Although there can be other reasons for a missed period, pregnancy is the most common cause. You should be able to get a fairly reliable test result if you wait for six weeks after your last period or roughly two weeks after the date you expected the period that did not materialize.

The other common symptoms of pregnancy include nausea, sickness, feeling tired, needing to urinate much more often than usual, swollen and tender breasts, constipation, disliking foods that you have previously liked, and wanting foods that you normally don't particularly care for. One of the reasons that many women do not at first realize that they are pregnant is that some of the symptoms, such as feeling tired, needing to urinate more often, swollen and tender breasts and constipation, are also signs of an approaching menstrual period. However, it is sometimes possible to recognize pregnancy by the *absence* of the twitchiness and anxiety experienced by some women in the syndrome known as premenstrual tension. Early morning sickness provides another clue.

The typical sickness of pregnancy starts at around the sixth week and continues in many women until about 14 weeks. Some women experience nausea and sickness throughout pregnancy, but this is rare. Pregnant women often experience sickness in the early morning and then not for the rest of the day; however, some feel sick all day for the first few weeks. Feeling or being sick, incidentally, are terms not normally used by doctors as they can lead to confusion: *feeling* sick is referred to as nausea and *being* sick is called vomiting. Neither of these conditions indicate that there is anything amiss with the pregnancy; however, if you are vomiting regularly and profusely (more than twice a day), you should seek your doctor's advice without delay.

When you are pregnant, you may find that you need to urinate more often than usual. This happens because of the increased pressure upon your bladder, and because of alterations in muscle tone due to hormonal changes. It tends to occur in the first eight to nine weeks of pregnancy; after this the uterus, containing the fetus, moves upwards, thus relieving the pressure to some extent. Some women, however, find that they need to pass water constantly throughout pregnancy. It is also not uncommon to be somewhat incontinent, so that when you laugh or cough, you involuntarily pass water. Needless to say, this can be very embarrassing. There are two things you can do: wear a pad when you go out, and perform the exercises described in the previous chapter designed to strengthen the muscles of the pelvic and abdominal area. These muscles become more and more stretched during pregnancy and the floor of the pelvis softens, both factors which contribute to this involuntary leaking.

You may notice that your breasts are rather tender and appear to be swollen at around six to eight weeks after your last monthly period. You may also notice changes in the nipples (they become harder and are extremely sensitive) and the areolae, the pinkish-brown area of the breasts. They may become browner in color and small white spots may become more pronounced. Breast tenderness disappears after eight weeks into the pregnancy.

Constipation is one of the irritating facts of pregnancy and it of course contributes to a feeling of bloatedness. Do not take drugs for this: Follow instead the guidelines for a sensible diet described in the previous chapter.

TESTING FOR PREGNANCY

Around the time that the common symptoms of pregnancy occur, usually at six weeks after your last monthly period, a pregnancy test can confirm that you are probably pregnant. However, many early pregnancies do not "take" and result in miscarriage. If there is a reason to be concerned about the viability (potential life) of a fetus, your doctor may recommend an ultrasound. By the sixth or seventh week of pregnancy, ultrasound can ascertain the location of pregnancy, visualize the fetal heartbeat and determine the number of fetuses.

Negative pregnancy urine test results are much less reliable and you should not assume that you are not pregnant until you receive a second negative result, or until you have a blood test. (If, after a second negative result, you have still not had a period, you should consult your doctor.)

Obtaining a pregnancy test

You can arrange to have a pregnancy test done by your doctor, by a hospital or by a family planning clinic. Alternatively, you can buy an over-the-counter kit and test yourself.

All these tests are based on detecting and measuring the amount of HCG—one of the specific pregnancy hormones excreted in the urine. It is also possible to measure HCG in the blood. The amount of HCG in a woman's body normally doubles every two to three days in the first six weeks of pregnancy. Pregnancy tests always suggest you use or supply an early morning urine sample, because HCG is present in the bladder in its greatest concentrations in the morning.

How pregnancy tests work

The common feature to all pregnancy tests is, currently, the measurement of HCG. They work, typically, according to the principle of agglutination, described below. A few tests work on the principle of color change.

The urine sample is mixed with an anti-HCG substance. If the woman is pregnant, the urine will contain HCG which neutralizes the anti-HCG. The mixture is added to a suspension of particles coated with HCG. If the woman is pregnant, there will be no reaction because the anti-HCG has been neutralized. If the woman is not pregnant, the particles are agglutinated (the particles clump together and cannot be separated) by the unfixed (non-neutralized) anti-HCG.

More recently, colorimetric tests based on color changes have become widely used.

How reliable are pregnancy tests?

Pregnancy tests sound straightforward in theory, but in practice a number of factors can make them produce unreliable results. Firstly, some 5–10 % of normal, non-pregnant women have some detectable but low levels of HCG in the body anyway and this could produce a positive result to the untrained eye. This poses a problem only with home pregnancy kits; medical staff, using more sophisticated techniques, would know that the levels of HCG are not consistent with those seen in pregnancy. Secondly, women are occasionally prescribed HCG for medical reasons; this could also give a false-positive test result. Thirdly, reliability of such tests depends very much on the time in relation to the last monthly period that they are performed. If they are performed earlier than six weeks after the last monthly period, the chances of receiving a misleading result are much higher. Fourthly, any trace of blood or vaginal discharge (which are also forms of protein) in the urine sample can produce a false-positive result. In the context of pregnancy, receiving the wrong result can be more frustrating and upsetting than not having a result at all. Finally, certain hormonal problems can occasionally result in false-positive tests; thyroid and ovarian stimulating hormones, for example, are similar in structure to HCG.

With home pregnancy testing kits, other factors are known to produce wrong results. These include:

1. performing the test incorrectly
2. performing it correctly but reading the result incorrectly
3. performing the test correctly and reading the result correctly, but the reagent substance fails to function properly.

Early testing

The massive surges of HCG in pregnant women at the time of implantation of the embryo facilitate biochemical pregnancy testing. If the first test is negative, a second test may be needed in a few days, as the levels of HCG double every few days in the first six weeks of pregnancy. The level of HCG can be measured in a hospital laboratory and is assessed by experienced technicians. The mere presence of HCG does not necessarily and exclusively indicate the existence of a normal pregnancy.

One of the factors to confound such tests is the rate of what is known as pregnancy failure. It is accepted that some 15% of recognized pregnancies fail to come to term: In other words, spontaneous abortion (miscarriage) occurs. Some experts believe that the rate of pregnancy failure is actually very much higher—perhaps as high as 78% of all pregnancies. It is thought that a large number of pregnancies fail at a very early stage—within the first two or three weeks—before pregnancy has been presumed or recognized. If this is so, it would account in part for the small number of positive pregnancy tests in women who are subsequently found not to be pregnant. Such a high failure rate in human pregnancies would be consistent with long-held theories surrounding natural selection and survival of the fittest.

Complications

Although a pregnancy may not be normal and may either terminate spontaneously or have to be terminated, as in the case of ectopic pregnancy, HCG may nevertheless be produced in the woman's body. A blighted ovum, for example, will fail to develop, but HCG may still be produced. In some 1 in 2,000 women in western countries, what is known as hydatidiform mole develops. This is a type of tumor of the chorionic villi, part of the structure of the chorion which is the outer of the two membranes normally destined to surround the baby in the uterus. Many of the normal symptoms of pregnancy will exist and HCG will be produced in very large quantities. It is because of complications such as this, and the other problems in obtaining a reliable pregnancy test result, that such tests allow the presumption of normal pregnancy rather than the proof.

CONFIRMATION OF PREGNANCY

An ultrasound scan can be invaluable in determining the definite existence of a pregnancy and the age of the embryo. A scan can be performed after six to seven weeks of suspected pregnancy; once you see the embryonic or fetal heartbeat, you need have no more doubts.

Pregnancy can also be detected by physical examination after about seven weeks, and if there is any doubt, an ultrasound scan can resolve the question.

YOUR DELIVERY DATE

The age of the embryo, and therefore the date at which you are likely to give birth, can be calculated from hospital HCG tests as accurately as by working it out from your last monthly period or by ultrasound. Knowing the age of the embryo/fetus is now essential for efficient prenatal care and the medical management of labor and birth. Management of complications in late pregnancy depends on accurate dating, so it is important to see a doctor or midwife as soon as you suspect that you are pregnant, to take advantage of the technology that medical science now has to offer. Many of these tests can identify problems and complications at such an early stage that they can be resolved with no further threat to the pregnancy. Very serious complications, such as severe preeclampsia (see p. 42), which can lead to the mother having fits and the life of the baby being seriously threatened, can be completely avoided by early identification of the risk, simply by measuring blood pressure regularly, close medical supervision and appropriate treatment.

Delivery dates are often calculated wrong, usually because the pregnant woman has confused the date of the last monthly period or has presented herself too late for accurate dating—in other words, after 16 weeks. If you are hoping to become pregnant, do make a note of the day each period starts and stops until you think that you may be pregnant. If you have the date of the first day of your last period, add seven days to it and then add nine calendar months in order to calculate the "due date." Alternatively, if you are certain that you know the date of ovulation, add 268 days to it; or add 282 days from the first day of your last period. Most people think of pregnancy lasting nine months, which, very roughly, it does. Doctors, however, need to be more precise and will always discuss your pregnancy with you in terms of weeks, rather than months. There are three distinct phases to pregnancy—the three trimesters. The first runs from 0–13 weeks, the second from 14–28 and the third from 29–40. Pregnancy is commonly assumed to last for 40 weeks; in practice, however, many women go into labor a week or two early and many others do so a week or so later than the 40th week.

INITIATING PRENATAL CARE

As you will see from the following chapters, precision concerning dates is valuable. If you have any reason to believe that your dates may be wrong, be sure to mention this to each doctor who sees you and explain by how many days or weeks you think the calculated dates could be wrong. All medical decisions in a woman's pregnancy depend on a knowledge of the age of the growing baby. Early prenatal care is an essential part of the safe medical management of your pregnancy, and is the subject of the next chapter.

5. The Initial Visit

Once you have decided where to go for care and have made your initial appointment, it is time to initiate care. The following discussion covers what to expect at the initial visit. It also explains what types of tests may be ordered early in your pregnancy to detect problems or confirm that all is going well.

The groundwork for your prenatal care is laid at your initial visit to the doctor or midwife you have chosen. One of the most important decisions you will need to make is whom to see for prenatal care and where you will have your baby.

If you are undecided about where to seek prenatal care, it is a good idea to interview prospective doctors or midwives. Many providers of maternity services will provide a free consultation or interview for prospective parents. These are important issues to consider:

1. Where are the offices?
2. What are the office hours? If you work, be sure the location and hours will enable you easily to keep appointments.
3. Where does the doctor/midwife or medical practice deliver?
4. What are the fees, and when are they collected? Some practices wait until after delivery to collect from your insurance company; others will expect you to pay their fee in advance.
5. Does the practice accept your insurance?
6. If it is a group practice, how do the doctors and midwives rotate delivery duty? Will you know in advance who will

deliver your baby, and if not will you meet each member of the group?

7. If it is a solo practice, who provides backup for the practitioner's vacations or illnesses? Can you make arrangements to meet the backup person?

THE FIRST PRENATAL VISIT

The first person you will speak with when you visit your doctor for the first time will probably be an office nurse. The nurse will request standard information from you, including:

- your name, address and telephone number at home and at work
- your date of birth
- your occupation
- your former name, if you have changed your name
- your birthplace
- your marital status
- your religion
- your family doctor's address and telephone number
- your partner's name, address, telephone number and occupation
- your next of kin, their relationship to you, their address and telephone number
- the language you speak

The doctor or nurse will then go on to medical matters. He or she will make a note of previous pregnancies as follows:

- date, place, length of pregnancy, birth weight and any problems that may have occurred during pregnancy, labor or in the immediate postnatal period

Turning to your current pregnancy, you will be asked:

- the date of your last menstrual period and whether or not you are certain of the date
- your estimated delivery date (EDC, or expected date of confinement)
- whether or not your periods are regular (which would affect the calculation of your EDC)
- whether or not you have had any vaginal bleeding since your last period (this could indicate a number of different conditions)
- whether or not you have been taking a contraceptive pill within three months of the last menstrual period (which could affect the calculation of your EDC)

PAST ILLNESSES AND OPERATIONS

The next set of questions concern your medical history. You will be asked if you have had any operations, blood transfusions, broken bones and so on. You will also be asked if you have ever suffered from anemia, jaundice, hepatitis and other conditions which could have a bearing on your health in pregnancy, and you will be asked if anyone in your family has suffered from diabetes, epilepsy, and a number of other diseases that tend to run in families, including Huntington's Chorea, hemophilia, Tay-Sachs disease, thalassemia and sickle cell disease. You will, in addition, be asked if you have had rubella (German measles) and if you have been in recent contact with anyone suffering from it.

INITIAL TESTING

You will then have a number of routine tests. Everyone has these and there is no need to be alarmed by the number of tests:

Blood tests
Tests, from a sample of blood taken from your arm, will be carried out:

- to determine your blood group (in case you later need a blood transfusion) and to determine whether you are rhesus positive or rhesus negative
- to determine your blood count, in case you are anemic
- to make sure you are immune to rubella
- to check your blood sugar level
- to ensure that there is no sign of hepatitis B, if you are at risk
- to detect blood disorders such as sickle cell disease and thalassemia, if you are at risk
- to check for AIDS antibodies if you are in a high-risk group for the disease, or if you ask for the test. People with a high risk of contracting AIDS include those who have had numerous lovers or a bisexual partner, anyone who shares a needle to inject illegal drugs intravenously and anyone who has had a blood transfusion anywhere in the world during the mid-to-late 1980s. It is not compulsory to undergo an AIDS test, but may become so. The results of an AIDS test will be kept confidential and separately from your medical record, so that staff do not know until labor starts, which is when it matters
- to determine if you have signs of syphilis

Urine tests
You will be asked to provide a small specimen of urine taken in the early morning *before* you drink anything.

· The specimen is checked principally for protein, sugar, bilirubin level, and salts and blood in the urine, in order to detect a number of conditions which could affect your pregnancy. Such conditions include kidney disease, diabetes and infections in the urinary tract, such as cystitis.

In order for this test to be performed as efficiently as possible, you need to provide the hospital with what is known as a mid-stream urine sample (MSU). To obtain this you need first to pass a little urine into the toilet, then contract your muscles for a couple of seconds to halt the flow and allow some of the remaining urine to pass into the specimen cup, and then finish passing water. In this way the hospital laboratory will have a sample of urine in mid-stream.

Pap smear

As part of the routine testing you will be given a Pap smear, unless you have had one within the last year. This is a routine investigation recommended for all women every one to two years regardless of whether or not they are pregnant. Ideally, you should have a smear before you are pregnant as it is then easier to treat any problems. A Pap smear is performed in order to detect any changes in the cells of the cervix at an early stage, before such changes can develop into cervical cancer. If precancerous changes in the cervix are picked up at an early stage, the disease can usually be treated successfully. Cervical cancer, when not treated or treated much too late, can be fatal.

A cervical swab, as well as a smear, is performed if you have herpes or you have had it in the past. It may be necessary in this case for the hospital to take a swab from the cervix weekly for about a month before your estimated delivery date. If the herpes virus is detected, you may be recommended for Cesarean, rather than vaginal, delivery in order to prevent the baby becoming infected with the virus as it moves downwards during birth from the uterus to the vagina. The virus does not penetrate the sac surrounding the baby during the pregnancy. Having a Cesarean, therefore, protects the baby from the contact that would cause it to contract the virus.

CVS or Amniocentesis

If you are considering having genetic testing, you should raise the question at your initial visit. It will probably be raised with you if you are considered to be in an "at risk" group. CVS (see pp. 44) is usually done at the tenth week, and amniocentesis (see Chapter 7) at 15–16 weeks, so it is important to discuss these tests early to allow time for counseling and scheduling.

PHYSICAL EXAMINATIONS

At one of your initial visits, you will also have a physical examination, at which the following are noted on your records: height, weight, blood pressure, lung function and condition of your teeth. You will also have a breast examination to detect any lumps. This routine check need not alarm you. Many women have slightly lumpy breasts, particularly if they have not had any children before. Of those who do have a lump, some 90% have simple, benign lumps; the remaining 10% may have malignant growths but, provided these are detected early, they can now be removed in a simple operation that leaves the breast intact.

You will also probably have an internal exam, in which a doctor examines manually your pelvic organs—in other words, your uterus, ovaries, cervix and vagina. Some women regard this type of examination as invasive and unpleasant, while others see it as a routine check. In any event, it does not take long and does not cause discomfort if performed by an experienced and considerate doctor.

Provided that all your test results and examinations are satisfactory, you will not need to visit the office for another four weeks. You may be given an alphafetoprotein test at the 16th week, and you may be offered amniocentesis (see Chapter 7). Pregnant women are usually advised to attend the prenatal clinic every four weeks until the 28th week of pregnancy; once every two weeks for the next eight weeks (until the 36th week) and from that time once a week until labor starts.

TEST RESULTS

Many, many tests are performed on every pregnant woman and it may not be surprising, therefore, that you are not told, "Yes, that's fine," to each test. It is quite possible that you may be given the result only if it merits a follow-up or a decision to be made. If you would like to know your results, however, there is no reason not to ask.

WHAT ARE ALL THE TESTS FOR?

You may be wondering by now why every pregnant woman undergoes so many tests and investigations. The principal reason is that all tests and investigations are done to eliminate the possibility of some complication, which, if allowed to continue untreated, could cause serious problems later in pregnancy or during labor. Your blood pressure, for example, is taken to make sure that it is not too high; if it is too high, it is easily brought down with tablets that do no harm to the developing baby. High blood pressure, which is more common if you are very overweight, is a typical sign of pre-eclampsia. Eclampsia is a condition that is peculiar only to pregnancy and if undetected can prove life-threatening to the pregnant woman and the baby; in its fully developed stage it is characterized by high blood pressure, severe headaches and fits. The signs of pre-eclampsia are high blood pressure, swelling of the ankles and hands, protein in the urine and sudden weight gain. This condition is one of the reasons for repeated blood pressure measurements, urine tests and weighing at each prenatal visit.

Traditional medical practitioners have often been strongly criticized for their apparent failure to practice preventative medicine. Prenatal care, however, is the best and most widespread example of preventative medicine. This is probably the only area of medical expertise in which doctors are expected and encouraged to anticipate problems in their patients and to treat them promptly and appropriately. The success of prenatal care is best measured by the decreasing death rates in mothers and babies compared with those rates of 50 and 100 years ago. It is now ten times safer than it was 100 years ago to have a child. The tragedy of prenatal care is that many women fail to obtain regular care due to economic constraints. This can result in enormous economic and social costs due to maternal and infant health problems which could have been prevented.

You may have heard of pregnancy diabetes and pre-eclampsia, but there may be other tests for things you have not heard of before. The rest of this chapter deals with some of the tests and conditions that may be unfamiliar to you. You will not be tested for rare conditions unless you are thought to be an "at-risk" individual, for reasons of your family medical history, your own medical condition, your racial origin or your lifestyle. See also pages 157–58.

CONDITIONS AND TESTS

anemia

anencephaly (see neural tube defects

blood sugar

chorionic villus sampling

chromosomal defect

cord blood sampling

cystic fibrosis

diabetes: established (classic) diabetes; gestational or pregnancy diabetes

Down's syndrome (pre-eclampsia)

epilepsy

established diabetes (see diabetes)

gestational diabetes (see diabetes)

hemophilia

hepatitis

Huntington's Chorea

hydrocephaly (see neural tube defects)

jaundice

kidney disease

muscular dystrophy

neural tube defects

pre-eclampsia

pregnancy or gestational diabetes (see diabetes)

rhesus factor

rubella (German measles)   Tay-Sachs disease
sickle cell disease   thalassemia
spina bifida (see neural tube
  defects)

Anemia

It is fairly common for women to become anemic during pregnancy, and this is a condition that can be treated easily by taking iron supplements. Since anemia can result in loss of oxygen to the baby, it is very important that it be treated. Anemia is detected by checking the hemoglobin levels in your blood, by means of a simple blood test; hemoglobin is responsible for carrying oxygen around your body and therefore to the growing baby. If hemoglobin levels are low, the baby is not receiving sufficient oxygen for healthy growth. There is nothing to be gained by taking more iron than you are prescribed because any surplus will be excreted and will also cause constipation. But if the condition is left untreated, not only does the baby receive insufficient oxygen, but your heart has to work harder to supply the baby with the oxygen it does receive, which makes you tired. It is also very important not to be in labor in an anemic state because there would be little reserve should you lose blood or require an operation.

Blood sugar

You may hear blood sugar referred to as blood glucose and you may be told, or see on your record, that you are to have a glucose tolerance test. The blood's level of glucose is the body's most important source of energy. However, if it is persistently high, it can indicate the presence of diabetes, which, in turn, indicates a lack of insulin, the hormone that makes use of glucose or sugar and converts it in the body to energy. Very overweight women often have high glucose levels. This condition is not healthy, particularly in pregnancy, and such women must be carefully supervised. (High blood sugar often leads to high urine sugars and this is one of the reasons urine is tested regularly.)

Chorionic villus sampling

This is a test normally carried out between the eighth and tenth week to detect inherited diseases—genetic defects—in the fetus. Chorionic villus sampling can identify the sex of the embryo and the existence of Down's syndrome and inherited disorders such as hemophilia, muscular dystrophy, cystic fibrosis, sickle cell disease and thalassemia. It cannot test for, or detect, spina bifida (neural tube defect). This technique is still being developed and is not offered to all women, nor by all hospitals.

Its advantages are that it can identify serious diseases at an early stage, thus providing the woman with the opportunity of an early termination of pregnancy if she wishes it. (Abortions are better performed early, before the 13th week, rather than later [this is explained in more detail in Chapter 7].) The disadvantage of this technique is that it is less accurate than amniocentesis, may be more likely to cause miscarriage, and does not test for spina bifida, which amniocentesis can do.

In the technique, which takes about 15 minutes, a narrow tube is passed into the uterus (either through the vagina or through the abdomen) to the outer sac surrounding the baby, known as the chorion. A small sample of the floating tendrils of the chorion, the villi, can be sucked into the tube and analyzed for information about the baby's genes. Ultrasound is used throughout the procedure to locate precisely the chorion and the villi.

Because of the hazards of miscarriage with this technique, it is unlikely that you will be offered it unless you are over 35 years old or your family has a history of one of the diseases that this test is able to identify. It cannot be performed after the 11th week as the chorion develops into the placenta and the chorionic villi disperse. The alternative is percutaneous umbilical blood sampling (PUBS) (see page 47) or amniocentesis at around the 16th week (see Chapter 7).

Chromosomal defect

A chromosomal defect is a defect of the chromosomes. Everyone has 23 pairs of chromosomes. The human body is made up of a large number of cells, each of which contains a nucleus. Each nucleus contains a set of 23 pairs of chromosomes. Our chromosomes contain the many genes which determine all the characteristics of an individual. In women, there are 22 pairs of chromosomes plus the sex chromosomes, XX. In men, the 23 pairs are made up, again, of 22 pairs plus the sex chromosomes, XY. When sperm and egg come together, the fertilized egg will consist of 23 unpaired chromosomes from the father and 23 unpaired chromosomes from the mother; these will pair off to produce the normal 23 pairs. This means to say that it is possible, although not automatic, that any defect in the parents' chromosomes may be passed on to the baby.

The chromosomes are grouped in pairs and this means that it is possible for someone to be a carrier of a disease, without developing it, because the disease-producing effects of the chromosome are counteracted by its opposite healthy number. However, if both parents are carriers, neither of them having developed the disease, a child may inherit the defective chromosome and develop the disease. This will happen if the child receives the defective chromosome from both parents. When it was present in the parents, it was counteracted by the healthy member of the pair and the disease, therefore, did not appear. However, now that the child has two defective genes, there is no healthy member of the pair to block the effect. This is known as a *recessive* gene disorder because it will only show itself when the two members of the pair are both defective. Cystic fibrosis is an example of a recessive gene disorder.

In recessive gene disorders, such as cystic fibrosis (the most common chromosomal defect seen in white races), four possibilities exist. Remember that the egg and the sperm from the parents each contain *one* of each member of the parents' pairs of chromosomes. The four possibilities are that:

1. neither parent donates the defective gene. In other words, of the chromosome pair responsible for the defect, it is the healthy half, in both cases, which passes into the sperm and egg. The child will, therefore, not inherit the disease.
2. the mother passes on the defective gene but the father donates the healthy half of the pair. The child will therefore become a carrier but not develop the disease. If the child in its adult life has children, it may pass on the defect.
3. the father passes on the defective gene but the mother does not. The outcome for the child will be that same as in 2, above.
4. both parents pass on the defective gene and the child will, therefore, receive a double dose, and develop the disease.

It can be said, therefore, that when both parents are carriers of a recessive gene disorder, the child has a 2 in 4 chance of being a carrier, a 1 in 4 chance of developing the disease, and a 1 in 4 chance of being normal.

In disorders in which the defective gene is dominant, if both parents have one defective gene each, the child has a 75% chance of inheriting the defect and also of developing the disorder. If one or both parents have two defective genes, the child has a 100% chance of inheriting the defect and the disorder. However, usually only one parent has the disease and the child, therefore, has a 1 in 2 chance of inheriting the defect and developing the disorder. If one parent has the defect, there are two possibilities for the child:

1. the defective member of the pair is passed on and because it is dominant the child will develop the disease;
2. the healthy member of the pair is passed on and the child will therefore not develop the disease.

Cord blood sampling or percutaneous umbilical blood sampling (PUBS)

This technique involves taking blood from the umbilical cord and analyzing the baby's blood cells, using much the same method as amniocentesis (see Chapter 7). Both techniques make use of ultrasound to guide the needle to the correct location. PUBS can be performed late on in the pregnancy, from the 18th week, to determine the condition of the baby and identify inherited disorders like those detected with amniocentesis. The advantage of PUBS is that results are available within a week, while amniocentesis usually means a wait of a month. PUBS may be used if a late ultrasound scan appears to indicate that something is amiss or if the alphafetoprotein test (see Chapter 7) reveals a level of protein that is too low. Like amniocentesis, cordocentesis carries a 1% chance of causing miscarriage. Rhesus negative women will require an injection of anti-D antibody after this test in case any fetal cells are disturbed, which would increase the risk of antibodies developing (see Rhesus factor, pages 52–53).

Cystic fibrosis

This is the most common chromosomal defect seen in the Caucasian population (white races). It is a single gene *defect*, as opposed to an *absence* of part of a gene as in Down's syndrome. Cystic fibrosis is a rare hereditary defect affecting many different glands, including the mucous glands of the bronchi, the sweat glands and the digestive glands. It leads to severe digestive problems, difficulty with breathing, lung infections and, because the sweat glands are adversely affected, a tendency to heatstroke.

If both parents are carriers, there is a 1 in 4 chance of a child inheriting the gene from both parents and developing the disease, although neither parent may have developed the disease (see *Chromosomal defect* on pages 45–46). Nearly half of all children so affected die before they reach the age of 20.

Cystic fibrosis can be tested for by DNA probe before conception with 85% accuracy. Alternatively, in pregnancy, the disorder can be tested for by amniocentesis or by chorionic villus sampling. Amniocentesis will identify 90% of affected fetuses, with a 5–6% false-positive rate. The test is therefore not sufficiently specific to offer to low-risk individuals.

Diabetes

There is no reason why a diabetic woman may not bear a child but she will need very careful medical supervision so that her blood sugar and insulin levels are rigidly controlled. Because of this the diabetic woman may expect to attend prenatal clinics more frequently than the nondiabetic woman, and to have repeated blood and urine tests. You can now test your own blood sugar with a small kit, available through your doctor's office, hospital or pharmacy. All diabetic women will be positively encouraged to accept hospital prenatal care and a hospital delivery. (This type of diabetes is commonly referred to as established diabetes, classic diabetes or full-blown diabetes. See also Gestational or Pregnancy diabetes, following.)

Down's syndrome
This is a genetic error which causes a condition in which both physical and mental impairment may exist. It can be inherited and it can also occur sporadically. The chances of a child being born with Down's syndrome rise sharply with the mother's age: for example, a 20-year-old woman has a chance of 1 in 2,000 of bearing a child so affected and a 40-year-old woman as a 1 in 100 chance.

Down's syndrome children tend to have a somewhat flat face, with a vertical fold of skin at the inner edge of the eye. The physical and mental impairment varies, ranging from fairly mild to severe mental retardation.

Eclampsia
See Pre-eclampsia.

Epilepsy
This condition is inherited by some 2% of children who have an epileptic parent. The epileptic woman will need very careful medical management for a safe pregnancy and delivery. Anticonvulsant drugs, used to control the fits typical of epilepsy, all cause folic acid (vitamin B12) depletion and supplements must therefore be taken. Such anticonvulsants also cause a low risk of abnormality, but this risk to the baby is much lower than the risk would be from its mother's epileptic fits, which could prove life-threatening.

Gestational (pregnancy) diabetes
This is a form of diabetes that occurs in pregnancy and clears up soon after the birth. It is just as hazardous as established diabetes (see above), and such cases have to be managed very carefully. Complications include still births, pre- eclampsia, urinary infections, excessively large babies (making vaginal deliveries very difficult unless performed some two to three weeks before term by induction (see Chapter 10)). Close fetal monitoring is certain to be recommended (discussed in Chapters 9 and 11). The baby of a diabetic mother is more likely to develop respiratory and other problems, and for these reasons the baby may be moved to an infant special-care unit directly after the birth. There is no reason, these days, why a diabetic woman or one with pregnancy diabetes may not give birth to a healthy child, provided that specialist

medical staff are on hand to assist. A home birth would present an unacceptably high risk to the baby.

Hemophilia

This rare chromosomal disorder is usually inherited only by men, but women can be carriers, passing it on to male children. If a woman has established that she is a carrier before she becomes pregnant, by means of DNA testing, she can have tests such as chorionic villus sampling (between the eighth–tenth weeks of pregnancy) or amniocentesis (at about the 16th week) to determine the sex of the fetus. If one of those tests indicated that the fetus was male, and thus stood a 50–50 chance of inheriting hemophilia, the woman could elect for a termination of pregnancy (see Chapter 7).

Hemophilia is a difficult disease for the child and his parents to manage. Essentially, the child's blood lacks the clotting factor and, therefore, if the child sustains the slightest injury involving bleeding, prolonged and uncontrolled bleeding results. This means that the child is prevented to some extent from leading a normal life: The rough and tumble of family life and the school playground are denied to the hemophiliac boy. Many die in childhood.

Hemorrhage

In pregnancy, hemorrhaging means bleeding from the vagina. By definition, this is known, if it is before the 24th week, as a threatened abortion; after the 24th week and before delivery it is known as antepartum hemorrhage. After delivery it is known as postpartum hemorrhage. Antepartum hemorrhage can be divided into two types: (1) incidental bleeding, which could come from the cervix or a polyp, for example, and which represents no danger to mother or baby; (2) placental bleeding, which may threaten mother and/or child (see placenta previa and placental abruption in Chapter 10). If the placenta is bleeding because it has become detached, the mother's blood cells are lost and this leads to severe bleeding. Additionally, the baby cannot receive the oxygen upon which its life depends as the placenta is no longer attached to the mother.

Hepatitis

This is an acute viral infection of the liver. Both types of the disease, hepatitis A, and hepatitis B, can be very serious indeed. Hepatitis B, the more dangerous of the two, can be transmitted to the fetus who can then become a carrier. Many but not all doctors screen for hepatitis B exposure. Both the liver and the kidneys are under additional strain during pregnancy, as they have to cope not only with the mother's waste products but the baby's as well. At-risk women include those with jaundice (a sign of hepatitis), those who have traveled recently to an area where the disease is endemic (such as India and Africa), those with a bisexual partner, and those illegal drug users who share needles to inject intravenously. It is also possible, though rare, to contract the disease as a result of receiving a transfusion of contaminated blood. Women with hepatitis will be treated by staff who will take special precautions to avoid the risk of spreading the infection.

Huntington's Chorea

This debilitating chromosomal disorder is, fortunately, very rare. The disease causes impairment in speech, walking and hand movements. These are accompanied by severe mental deterioration, which usually requires hospitalization on a permanent basis. The disease usually proves fatal within about 15 years of its first appearance. Huntington's Chorea does not usually appear until middle age, which means that a woman may already have had children before she realizes that she has inherited it.

The hereditary risk is 50–50, so there is a reasonable chance that the child will not inherit it (see *Chromosomal defect*, on pages 45–46). If you know that someone in your family or wider family (including grandparents, aunts and uncles) had or has the disease, and you are not already pregnant, it is now possible, by DNA testing, to establish whether or not you are a carrier. If you are not, you need have no fears about having a baby.

If you are pregnant, you will have to choose between your desire to have children and the knowledge that that child stands a 50% chance of developing the disease in its middle age. In addition, you will have to consider how you will be able to look after your children if you yourself develop the disease in middle age, when your children may still be quite young.

Jaundice

This is rare in pregnancy but it is an important sign in that it can indicate hepatitis (see on page 449–50). Jaundice may be worsened by pregnancy as a result of the greater workload upon the mother's liver. It can be caused by an obstruction of the biliary tract—gallstones, for example—leading to incomplete excretion and a consequent buildup of waste products which causes the typical yellow coloration of jaundice, seen in the whites of the eyes and the skin. A second cause of jaundice is the body breaking down too many blood cells, and a third is the malfunctioning of the liver (as in hepatitis and disease of the liver).

There is also a type of jaundice specific to pregnancy, which usually appears in the last trimester (weeks 29–40) and clears up soon after delivery of the baby. It is caused by the hormonal changes of pregnancy which lead to a blocking of the normal excretory processes.

Kidney disease, infections

One of the signs of kidney infection, common in pregnancy, is the appearance of protein in the urine, and this is one of the reasons that regular urine tests are made during pregnancy. Kidney infections are usually combined with sharp pain in the lower abdominal area and the groin, together with a raised temperature. Infections such as cystitis are more common in pregnancy and during this time such infections can travel up from the bladder to the outlet of the kidneys more easily.

Regular urine tests can help to identify pre-eclampsia, a complication of which is kidney damage if the pre-eclampsia remains undetected and untreated.

Apart from the special problems of temporary stress upon the kidneys during pregnancy, when the kidneys are working harder than normal in coping with both the mother's and the baby's waste products, there are also problems for the woman with established chronic kidney damage prior to pregnancy. Partly because of the increased workload upon the kidneys during pregnancy, but chiefly because it could lead to growth problems in the baby, such women should be under close medical supervision during pregnancy and labor in order to prevent gross damage or collapse of the kidneys.

Muscular dystrophy

This rare inherited chromosomal disorder usually affects boys, and only occasionally girls. Women, however, can be carriers and can therefore pass it on to their sons. As with hemophilia, early genetic testing, chorionic villus sampling or amniocentesis can detect the sex of the embryo in women who are known to be carriers and, if male, afford women the opportunity of terminating the pregnancy (see Chapter 7).

Muscular dystrophy is a wasting disease, in which the muscles of the body weaken and degenerate, for which there is no cure.

Neural tube defects

The neural tube is the spinal cord, "neuro" deriving from the Greek for nerve. The central nervous system is the brain and the spinal cord. If the baby's spinal cord fails to develop properly in the early weeks of pregnancy, congenital malformation or structural defects, known as neural tube defects, occur. These defects range from the very serious, such as the absence of a brain, to comparatively minor ones. Some 1–2 in every 1,000 babies are affected. Half will miscarry and some die soon after birth.

There are two categories of neural tube defects (NTDs): open NTDs and closed NTDs. In open NTDs, which comprise spina bifida and anencephaly (no brain), the cord has not closed properly, exposing the nervous tissue of the brain and/or the spinal cord—in other words, the skin is broken and the nerves are exposed. This means that the baby's spinal cord leaks the alphafetoprotein made in its liver out into the amniotic fluid, from which it crosses the placenta and enters the mother's bloodstream. This means that the AFP test (see Chapter 7) can detect these open neural tube defects. Open NTDs can also be tested for by amniocentesis (see Chapter 7).

Closed neural tube defects (which include hydrocephaly and meningomyelocele) can be detected only by detailed ultrasound scan because there is no leak of alphafetoprotein either in the amniotic fluid or blood. In other words, the spinal cord has failed to develop properly but it has closed. Hydrocephaly (water on the brain) may be apparent on a detailed ultrasound scan at 20 weeks (see Chapter 7): The ventricles of the brain may be dilated, with accompanying compression of the brain tissue. This leads eventually to a grossly enlarged head, spasticity and mental impairment.

It is possible for a baby to be affected by a combination of any of the four different neural tube defects, any one of which can be incompatible with normal life. But not all of them are. Although the worst affected babies may miscarry or die soon after birth, some survive. Some of the defects are treatable, others are not. Babies may suffer from severe mental and physical impairment or they may be only slightly affected—for example, with normal mental faculties and relatively minor physical handicap. If the defect affects the brain, mental impairment will invariably occur. If the problem occurs in the lower spine, the nerves are affected; this can lead to physical handicap which can include paralysis of the lower body and incontinence. (See also Chapter 7.)

Pre-eclampsia
This is one of the most common causes of fetal death before labor starts. It is the precursor to the very serious condition of convulsions in pregnancy, known as eclampsia, and can prove fatal. It is characterized by the development of high blood pressure, generalized swelling (face, ankles, wrists and sometimes all over the body) and by the appearance of protein in the urine. It usually manifests itself at around 30–34 weeks but can present itself earlier or later. It requires urgent referral to the hospital and admission to a prenatal ward. It is a common indication for early delivery either by induction or by Cesarean section. (See also pp. 36 and 42.)

Rhesus factor
When your blood test is carried out at the initial visit, your blood group will be noted (either A, AB, B or O) and so will the rhesus factor. Most people are rhesus positive, but some 15%, or 1 in 6 people, are rhesus negative. Rhesus- positive blood cells possess an antigen which can stimulate the production of antibodies to

fight alien blood cells. Rhesus-negative blood lacks this antigen. A problem arises in pregnancy only if you are rhesus negative; there are no problems if you are rhesus positive. If you are rhesus negative and the baby has the same blood *group* as you, but is rhesus positive, some of the blood cells that escape from its body into yours during pregnancy, and especially during the birth, will provoke your body to make antibodies to fight the alien cells and destroy them. This in itself does not harm you or, usually, the baby. However, a problem arises with second and subsequent pregnancies, if the fetus is again rhesus positive and the woman, of course, is rhesus negative. Because of the first pregnancy, the woman's body will now contain antibodies to fight and destroy rhesus positive cells. These antibodies can pass into the circulation of the second baby and break down its cells. This can result in serious problems, including stillbirth, severe anemia in the baby, heart failure, extreme jaundice, spasticity or mental impairment.

Because of the risk to second and subsequent babies, it is essential that rhesus-negative women are given anti-D injections during pregnancy after any invasive procedure such as chorionic villus sampling, PUBS and amniocentesis, and after the birth of their first child, and subsequent children, to destroy the antibodies.

If the woman is unlucky enough to develop antibodies, the danger to the current pregnancy will be that the antibodies cross the placenta from the mother and attach themselves to the baby's blood cells, which they then attack and destroy. This causes anemia and high bilirubin (a blood breakdown product) content in the baby. Anemia can lead to heart failure and death while the baby is still in the uterus. A high bilirubin level can lead to brain damage after the baby is born in the form of spasticity and mental impairment.

If antibodies are identified during pregnancy, they are measured and, according to the level, the baby will need PUBS or amniocentesis in order to measure the level of bilirubin in its blood and the drop in the blood count. It is possible to transfuse a baby (give the baby a blood transfusion) through the umbilical cord before birth and indeed even to exchange its blood while it is still in the uterus. After delivery it may be necessary to repeat the process of exchange transfusion.

There are no such problems if the rhesus-negative woman happens to have a rhesus-negative child, but this is less likely than having a rhesus-positive child, since only 1 in 6 of the population are rhesus negative.

Rubella (German measles)
Your blood is checked for immunity to the rubella virus at the initial visit because if you develop rubella (which used to be known as German measles) during pregnancy, particularly during the first

three months, perhaps before you even know you are pregnant, the baby may be severely affected. The virus can attack the baby's nervous system and its heart, and can cause deformity, handicaps such as deafness or blindness, miscarriage or stillbirth. Rubella is highly infectious, particularly at the time that any rash appears. However, it is also infectious for a week before and a week after any rash. The incubation period is between 14 and 21 days.

Rubella can exist in a very mild form and it is therefore difficult to diagnose. Women who catch it in the early stages of pregnancy may not realize it, mistaking the virus for a cold. Ideally, therefore, you should be checked for immunity to rubella before you attempt to become pregnant. If you are not immune, you can be vaccinated and then be re-checked to make sure that the vaccine has worked. It is important to have the rubella immunity test, even if you are certain that you have had rubella as a child, because rubella is a virus that has frequently been misdiagnosed, and because it is uncertain for how long immunity achieved in this way lasts.

Sickle cell disease
This is a hereditary chromosomal defect of red blood cells, commonly seen in people of African, West Indian and Asian origin and so all women of African, Afro-Caribbean and Asian descent should be tested. Many people of these origins may have the blood condition known as sickle cell trait, but this does not necessarily develop into sickle cell disease. However, if both the woman and her partner have the trait, the baby will have a 1 in 4 chance of developing the disease. Sickle cell disease is a form of anemia, in which the sufferer will have the signs and symptoms of anemia (see p. 44) together with an unusually large abdomen, because of an enlarged liver and spleen, with underdeveloped arms and legs. Other problems can include leg ulcers, passing blood in the urine, and painful and swollen joints.

Tay-Sachs disease
This rare disease, caused by a chromosomal defect which results in severe physical and mental handicap, is seen most frequently in Jews of central or Eastern European descent. When only one parent is a carrier, the child will not inherit the disease. However, if both parents are found to be carriers, the child can develop the disease. The carrier state, which does not cause ill health, can be identified quickly and easily by a blood test. At-risk individuals are advised to have this test before attempting to become pregnant. If someone is already pregnant, however, tests such as chorionic villus sampling or amniocentesis can identify the existence of the disease in the fetus and, if necessary, a termination of pregnancy would be offered (see Chapter 7).

Thalassemia

This is a rare and serious blood disorder, caused by a chromosomal defect. Thalassemia minor, the carrier state, is not serious in itself but if both parents have this, the child has a 1 in 4 chance of developing thalassemia major. The disease is usually seen in people from Mediterranean areas, Southeast Asia and India and Pakistan. Pre-pregnancy testing is advisable; if a woman is already pregnant, however, either chorionic villus sampling or amniocentesis can determine the existence of the disease in the fetus. If necessary, termination of the pregnancy can be considered (see Chapter 7).

If it is found, or suspected, that you have any of these conditions, or suspected that the fetus may have contracted one of them, you will be monitored more carefully and perhaps asked to attend the prenatal clinic at more frequent intervals than the customary four weeks (up to the 28th week). There are also certain conditions which, if detected, may compel you to consider the possibility of terminating this pregnancy. Such conditions include rubella contact, particularly in the first three months of your pregnancy; AIDS; and a family history of cystic fibrosis, Huntington's Chorea, sickle cell disease, Tay-Sachs disease and thalassemia. It may be advisable to have further tests before coming to a decision; these tests are the subject of Chapter 7.

If you are over 35 years of age, you may wish to have the amniocentesis test, described in Chapter 7, in order to eliminate any worry you may have about bearing a handicapped child. While this test cannot guarantee that you will give birth to a perfect baby, it can identify a number of serious defects, and therefore gives you the choice of whether or not to continue with the pregnancy.

Generally speaking, it is more than likely that your initial visit to the prenatal clinic will reveal nothing untoward and you will be able to leave the doctor's office with complete peace of mind, knowing that today's medical technology has eliminated many possible causes of worry for you.

ULTRASOUND

Ultrasound scans are known by a number of different names, which can be confusing: They may be referred to by different members of the medical and nursing staff as scans, ultrasounds, ultrascans, anomaly scans, realtime ultrasounds, realtime scans. All these terms mean the same thing: ultrasound scan. You may also hear of Doptone, Sonicaid or Doppler ultrasound, and these ultrasounds refer to ultrasounds using the Doppler effect (both described below). The "detailed" scan is the anomaly scan.

What ultrasound scans can do

In essence, these scans provide pictures of the fetus in the mother's body. Experts can tell from the pictures whether the baby is the correct size for its age; if it is growing normally; if there are twins (or more); and later in pregnancy it can be used again to check the baby's growth and to make sure the baby is in the correct position to deliver. Ultrasound is useful in calculating the estimated date of delivery, if an uncertainty over the date of the LMP exists, by revealing the size of the baby. If dates are certain, but the baby is either unusually small or unusually large, this can alert medical staff to a number of problems. For example, an unusually large baby may indicate diabetes in the mother, and may require a Cesarean delivery. A routine ultrasound, given at around the 18th week, can detect certain abnormalities and, if revealed, might merit an amniocentesis (see Chapter 7) or PUBS (described earlier in this chapter), or a termination if the fetus is clearly so severely abnormal as to be incapable of independent life. Ultrasound is the only way of discovering a twin or multiple pregnancy in its early stages and it is also the only way of obtaining positive proof of pregnancy in the first few weeks (as described in Chapter 4).

Pregnant women often will be given one or two ultrasound scans during their pregnancy. It is most important to have one at around 18 weeks. This scan will identify any developmental and structural abnormality in the fetus, which will not have been apparent at an earlier stage (such as the 12th week). These abnormalities include spina bifida, hydrocephaly and anencephaly, defects in the heart and kidneys, and hare lip.

If the other routine tests seem to indicate problems with the pregnancy, more ultrasound scans may be given. Such scans are particularly useful when certain medical conditions exist in the mother, such as high blood pressure, heart or kidney disease and diabetes. If the baby appears not to be growing well, the mother may have a series of serial scans (a scan once a month or more). This would also be the case if she was bleeding vaginally or if a twin or multiple pregnancy had already been identified (in order to make sure that all the babies were growing well). Those women who have had problems in previous pregnancies may also be offered more scans than the routine number. Medical practice varies to some extent from hospital to hospital and, of course, with each individual woman. It is impossible, therefore, to be precise about what is routine. Some doctors may not do any scans routinely, while others may do two or three. If you turn to the Table of Positive Risk Factors in Chapter 6, you will see what sort of things may make your doctor suggest an ultrasound scan.

Ultrasound is also used with amniocentesis, CVS and fetal blood sampling (see Chapter 7) in order that the needle may be guided to the precise spot. (See also pp. 99–100)

What happens when you have an ultrasound scan

You will be asked to drink one pint of water before the time of your appointment for the scan so that you have a full bladder. A full bladder causes the uterus, which normally lies behind the pelvic bones, to be pushed outwards. The uterus, containing the baby, can then be clearly seen on the scan.

You will be lying down for the scan, with your abdomen bared. Your skin has to be covered with a gel, as soundwaves cannot travel through air: The sensor, or probe, has to make a direct airtight contact with your skin. The probe is placed on your abdomen and you will almost immediately see a somewhat incomprehensible picture on the computer screen. The operator will point out what the patterns in the picture mean and show you your baby on the screen. You should be able to see the baby moving and you will see its heart beating from about the 6th-7th week. You will be able to *hear* the heartbeat from about the 12th–14th week with the Doptone auditory scan. Because the baby is so small at the time of your first scan (if it is done at anything up to 12 weeks), it will probably be impossible to see whether it is a girl or a boy. Even with later scans, it is very difficult, even for an experienced operator, to be sure whether the baby is a girl or boy. Recently, vaginal probes have been developed, and transvaginal ultrasound is widely used during pregnancy.

How ultrasound works

Ultrasound is sound that is a pitch higher than humans can hear. This sound can be directed into the body to produce echoes from the meeting points of different sorts of body tissue. Measurements of the echoes are returned to the computer terminal which can build up a moving picture on the screen. This type of ultrasound is known as realtime ultrasound and replaces an older type which could produce only static pictures.

Doppler ultrasound is a development of ultrasound which can detect waves of moving fluid because it can pick up moving structures, such as your blood, for example. The returning echo contains a change or shift in tone and this can be used to measure blood flow. It can, therefore, interpret the baby's heartbeat by monitoring blood flow. It is now thought that, as early as 24 weeks, it may be possible to predict those women who may develop pre-eclampsia on the basis of measuring their blood flow with Doppler ultrasound or machines using this principle This is still the subject of intense research and is carried out only on an experimental basis in selected cases.

Is ultrasound safe?

No one is prepared to say that ultrasound is definitely safe but there is currently no evidence to suggest that it is unsafe. However, doctors always restrict the number of ultrasound scans to what they consider is the minimum. Much of medicine has to observe what is known as the risk-benefit ratio: Medical practice is often a matter of assessing whether or not the advantages of a particular technique or drug regime outweigh the disadvantages. All the experts agree that the risks of ultrasound are very much lower than the benefits it offers and that the ratio is acceptable; that is, the risks of serious and undetected problems in pregnancy are considered to be much higher than any risks posed by ultrasound.

SCHEDULING THE NEXT VISIT

Your doctor or midwife will tell you when you need to return for your next visit. Probably you will not be asked to return for about four weeks; but if your first visit was late, the doctor or midwife may want you to come back sooner.

PART TWO

Weeks 14–28, the middle three months

6. The Prenatal Clinic

After reading the previous chapter, it should be clear that a wide array of tests and testing techniques can be used to determine a variety of risk factors in pregnancy: risks both to the mother and to the baby. Your prenatal care, from the time of the initial visit, will be determined by your medical history, your general medical condition and the outcome of the initial tests and examinations.

You will have seen from Chapter 5 that several options are open to you in your prenatal care and your delivery. This book is primarily concerned with the tests and technology of full hospital care and it therefore describes a large array of tests and techniques, many of which you will not receive if your pregnancy is identified as low-risk.

No one undergoes all the tests outlined in this chapter: Some women will have some of them if a positive risk factor has been identified. Remember that many pregnancies and two out of three births are quite straightforward.

Because this book is primarily concerned with high-tech pregnancy and birth, the rest of this chapter describes a program of prenatal care as would be found in either a hospital or obstetrician's office.

Provided that you have made your initial visit to the doctor during the first trimester of pregnancy (the first third, weeks 0–13) and no special risk reveals itself, you will probably be asked to return for your second visit to the prenatal clinic in four weeks. Your visits to the prenatal clinic are likely to proceed according to the schedule of routine tests, given on the following page. These amount to no more than the occasional blood test, measurement of blood pressure and weight, urine tests, and abdominal examination (all described in the previous chapter). All these constitute good, routine obstetric practice and are nothing to worry about.

AT THE INITIAL VISIT (12 WEEKS)

Blood tests:
blood count
blood group
rhesus antibody level test for rhesus-negative women (see below)
rubella immunity
venereal disease
hepatitis B
special blood test to identify sickle cell, thalassemia, Tay-Sachs,
    for those at risk
blood sugar
HIV antibodies, signifying possibility of AIDS (if required or
    advised in cases where AIDS is a potential risk)

Other tests
mid-stream urine sample
cervical smear (PAP smear)
cervical swab
urine test for drug profile (if indicated)

AT 16–18 WEEKS

ultrasound scan (see Chapter 5) to check size of baby and deter-
    mine due date
serum alphafetoprotein (see Chapter 7) or at any time between
    15 and 22 weeks to check the amount of protein, called
    alphafetoprotein, made in the baby's liver and detectable in
    the mother's blood
amniocentesis, for some women (see Chapter 7)

AT 24 WEEKS

rhesus antibodies check, if necessary

AT 28 WEEKS

blood test for anemia (in cases of previous anemia) and diabetes
    (only for high-risk women)
diabetes screening test
blood sugar (in some units)

AT 34 WEEKS

blood test for anemia and diabetes if urine sugar indicates the
    need for these tests
rhesus antibodies check, if necessary

Rhesus-negative women will be carefully monitored for the appearance of antibodies in the blood (signifying the existence of a rhesus positive baby, as described in the previous chapter) with blood tests at 24, 28 and 34 weeks.

EARLY IDENTIFICATION OF RISK FACTORS

If a positive risk is identified with your pregnancy you may be asked to return earlier for further tests or for examination, or both. Risk factors may be associated with your age, your menstrual cycle, your method of contraception before becoming pregnant, previous pregnancies and any associated complications, your health, any medical condition, your sexual history and medical problems arising during the pregnancy itself. If you are identified as "at risk," you may be offered more frequent ultrasound scans (described in the previous chapter) and you may also be offered amniocentesis (described in the next chapter). The positive risk factors, which will be noted on the medical record, are listed in the table on pages 65–72 together with their possible effects upon the woman and her baby and the action to be taken.

WHAT PRENATAL CARE CAN DO FOR YOU

This part of the book is concerned primarily with the middle trimester of pregnancy, weeks 14 to 28. However, in order to give a complete and coherent picture of the prenatal care now available to women, the Table of Positive Risk Factors covers the entire term of pregnancy. It is safe to say that most positive risk factors, if any exist, will be identified before week 28 and the appropriate treatment given.

Serious risks in pregnancy are not common; some of the risks are very rare indeed. Regular screening enables doctors to anticipate problems, to treat where appropriate and, when necessary, to arrange to have specialists in other fields present for the later stages of labor and the birth. In this way, a baby that needs emergency medical care, or an operation shortly after birth, can be cared for without delay. Quick and effective treatment often ensures the health of the baby. A premature baby, for example, can go directly into a special care baby unit for intensive care, while a baby with malformed or malfunctioning heart or lungs may be operated upon straight after delivery with complete success. Fifty or 100 years ago, such babies would have had little chance of survival. The importance of good prenatal care, and regular checkups, cannot be overemphasized.

Another aspect of prenatal care is the peace of mind that efficient medical assistance can provide. In the past, people who knew that a rare hereditary disease existed in their family often chose not to have children for fear that they were carriers of the disease and would pass it on. Testing before pregnancy and tests available during pregnancy now offer those "at risk" women the opportunity to bear a child without the disease. Some women may find that they are not carriers at all, or they may discover, as in the case of Tay-Sachs disease that because only one parent is a carrier, the child cannot inherit the disease.

If a prenatal test does identify the existence of a serious disease, that the child would be certain to inherit, a very difficult decision must be made. The parents must decide whether or not to terminate the pregnancy and to try again in a year or two for another child. This is discussed in the next chapter.

ASSESSING PROBLEMS

If a prenatal test identifies some sort of deformity or handicap in the child, it is important to discuss with an expert what may be involved. It can be quite difficult to identify the degree of handicap with prenatal tests and what that handicap may mean for the child and for you, the parents. Sometimes it is possible to assess the degree of handicap but not the extent of malfunction caused by that handicap.

Prenatal tests can identify, broadly speaking, four groups of handicap:

1. severe handicaps, such as absence of brain or deformed heart, which are not compatible with life (in other words, the child would die shortly after birth)
2. serious handicaps that are operable if known about before delivery, so the baby can receive an immediate emergency operation
3. handicaps which can in themselves be assessed but the degree of malfunction not anticipated for some time after birth
4. minor deformities, such as an extra finger, which can be removed in an operation

Some individuals resist testing, not wanting unpleasant news. But as medical knowledge advances, more can be done to correct some defects in utero. The medical staff should be willing to discuss the appropriate treatment (if available) with parents.

While it is true that not all defects or problems can be detected through testing, trusting to luck is not fair to you, your family or your child. Good prenatal care and efficient screening can take much of the worry out of pregnancy.

Table 6.1 POSITIVE RISK FACTORS

POTENTIAL RISK IN PRESENT PREGNANCY

Risk Factor	Potential Risk	Possible Action
Age less than 18	Anemia, pre-eclampsia, low-birth-weight baby, premature labor, baby's head too big to pass through mother's pelvis	Prenatal care in facility with nutritional and social services geared toward complex psychosocial needs of teenage pregnancy
35 or older	Placenta insufficient to nourish baby, hypertension (high blood pressure), large baby, gestational diabetes, genetic defects	Discuss amniocentesis, or chorionic villus sampling, assess fetal size by ultrasound, consider induction if baby late
Already have four or more children	More likely that the baby will be in difficult position for birth, placental insufficiency, anemia	Medical supervision of third stage of labor to prevent uterus from relaxing and so causing hemorrhage. Possibility of Cesarean for transverse lie (see pp. 110–111)
Uncertainty re date of LMP; contraceptive pill stopped within three months of LMP; menstrual cycle before LMP more than 30 days	Dates may be wrong and therefore EDC wrong	Early ultrasound scan to establish dates
IUD (coil) in place	Significant risk of miscarriage, premature breaking of waters, premature labor, infection, ectopic pregnancy	Immediate scan and appointment with consultant. Remove IUD if possible
Obesity	High blood pressure, gestational diabetes, large baby, birth injury, Cesarean section	Dietary counseling, ultrasound surveillance of fetal size, early diabetes testing
Vaginal bleeding after last period	Miscarriage, missed or incomplete abortion, ectopic pregnancy, hydatidiform mole (see Chapter 4), inaccurate dates	Immediate examination and scan, smear, blood group check, Rh immune globulin injection for rhesus negative women

Your previous pregnancies		
Previous stillbirth (from 20th week of pregnancy) or death of previous baby up to first 4 weeks of life	Risk of recurrence, preterm delivery, autoimmune disease (in which maternal antibodies may cause problems in baby or placenta)	Appointment with specialist. Regular scanning through the pregnancy to make sure baby is growing properly is very important. You may be screened for SLE and other autoimmune disease and your glucose tolerance may be checked. Possible induction of labor
Previous small baby	Low-birth-weight baby, small baby, placental insufficiency	Regular ultrasound scans to check growth, dietary counseling, increased bedrest, possible early induction of labor if current pregnancy affected
Previous large baby	Pregnancy diabetes, birth trauma for mother and baby, baby's shoulder may become lodged in the birth canal	Glucose tolerance test for diabetes, ultrasound scan to check growth and size of baby, possible induction of labor
Previous Cesarean, hysterotomy, or myomectomy (removal of fibroids)	Possible uterine rupture	Possible Cesarean. Report to hospital as soon as the start of labor is suspected
Two or more miscarriages before this pregnancy	Nonviable pregnancy—blighted ovum, see Chapter 3, another miscarriage, intrauterine growth, low birth-weight baby	Early scan (before the 12th week if possible), chromosomal blood tests, i.e., AFP, CVS or amniocentesis. Testing for autoimmune disease and SLE
In previous pregnancies: preterm labor (20–37 weeks), cervical stitch, late miscarriage or two or more terminations	Miscarriage, cervical incompetence, premature breaking of water bag, premature labor, mild genital infection	Possible bedrest, careful observation for preterm labor, SLE screening, possible cervical stitch
Congenital fetal abnormality in previous baby	Possible recurrence	Discussion with genetic counselor, scan at 18-20 weeks, chorionic villus sampling or amniocentesis if desired or medically indicated at 16 weeks, possible blood chromosome test for baby, termination if required

Antibodies in previous pregnancy which could cause harm to fetus, such as rhesus antibodies	Blood disorder of baby	Blood test from father as well as mother, full hospital care and repeated blood tests for rhesus antibody levels, referral to perinatologist if indicated. Baby may need intrauterine transfusions or early delivery
In previous pregnancies: eclampsia, pregnancy-induced hypertension or proteinuria (protein in urine, signifying kidney problems or predisposition to eclampsia)	Risk of recurrence, placental insufficiency	Specialized urine test, appointment with specialist to discuss problems. Ultrasounds to assess fetal growth
Severe bleeding after giving birth or manual removal of placenta (rather than being expelled naturally) in previous pregnancy	Possible recurrence	Full medical assistance in third stage of labor, possible blood donations in case maternal transfusion needed.
Very short labor (less than two hours) in previous pregnancy	Recurrence likely. Risk to baby, in home births, of delivery in transit to hospital	Go to hospital as soon as labor starts. Ideally, discuss with doctor possibility of going to hospital before labor starts. May be offered planned induction so that labor can be controlled
Long labor (more than 12 hours of active labor) in previous pregnancy	If pelvis too small, recurrence possible	Discuss birth plan with doctor, assessment of pelvis, possible Cesarean
Forceps in previous pregnancy	If pelvis too small, recurrence possible	As above
Postpartum depression after birth of previous baby	Recurrence	Specialist psychiatric consultation. Discuss with doctor the various forms of support available

Your own health and medical conditions

Relevant conditions include cardiac, kidney, hormonal, diabetic, blood disorders, cancers, gastrointestinal, respiratory, neurological, thromboembolic, psychiatric, genital infections. Any of these conditions may adversely affect the pregnancy or the pregnancy may make the condition from which you are suffering worse. Any of these conditions indicate that you should be attending prenatal clinic more frequently than once every four weeks, and you may also be seen by the relevant specialists as well as the consultant obstetrician. Other specific conditions include:

Uterine anomaly, including fibroids	Pain from fibroids. Presentation of baby other than head down. Obstructed labor	Preterm labor, possible bedrest, preterm labor treatment, ultrasounds to assess growth and posiion of fetus and fibroids.Removal may be recommended between pregnancies
Blood disorder (thalassemia or sickle cell disease or trait)	Baby may inherit the condition	Father to have blood test, possible CVS or amniocentesis, possible termination if desired
Family history of diabetes	Pregnancy diabetes	Test, if positive will be referred to diabetes specialist
Family history of congenital fetal abnormality	Possible risk of hereditary disease	Ultrasound screening for structural defects. Genetic counseling, chorionic villus sampling (if before 11th week) or amniocentesis at 16th week, chromosomal analysis of blood of mother and father, possible termination if desired
Smoking more than 10 cigarettes per day	Baby's growth retarded and powers of concentration and learning impaired, respiratory problems, much higher chance of cot death (Sudden Infant Death syndrome) in the baby	Stop smoking now. Ultrasounds to check baby's growth
Drinking more than 10 ounces of alcohol a week	Baby may be born with fetal alcohol syndrome, a pattern of physical and mental defects that include severe growth deficiency, heart defects, malformed facial features, a small head, abnormalities of coordination and movement, and mental impairment. Babies are born addicted to alcohol and may suffer withdrawal symptoms so that they are twitchy, restless, can't feed and won't thrive. They may have to be sedated to help them through the withdrawal phase	Cut down quickly. Pediatric specialist required at birth, long-term developmental followup of baby

Illegal drug taking by mother or partner	Baby born addicted, problems with giving pain relief in labor, baby's growth retarded. Placental abruption, preterm delivery	Screen for HIV and STD, developmental followup of baby
Number of different partners	Possibility of STDs and AIDS in mother and baby. Cogenital syphilis	As above
Anal intercourse	As above	As above
Bisexual partner	As above	As above
Risk of transmissible viral infection, such as hepatitis B and AIDS	Risk of infection to baby and to medical and nursing staff	Screen for HIV and STD; HBsAG, hepatitis vaccine and immune globulin for babies of carriers

Adverse social factors, housing problems and lack of fluency in English are also all identified as risk factors for the pregnant woman and a social worker should be asked to help the woman and her family through the pregnancy.

Risk factors identified at initial visit

Blood pressure 140/90 or more, taken after woman has been lying down for 5 minutes	Pregnancy hypertension (could lead to pre-eclampsia), placental insufficiency, complication of pre-eclampsia	Hospital care and more frequent visits to clinic, more urine tests and blood pressure measurements, fetal growth followed with ultrasound. Bed rest starting at 6 or 7 months
Protein in urine with normal blood pressure	Chronic kidney disease, bladder infection	Discussion with kidney specialist. More urine tests, and bacterial culture
Protein in urine, blood pressure raised	Pre-eclampsia	Possible immediate admission
Obesity (greater than 20 lbs. overweight)	Pregnancy hypertension, maybe leading to pre-eclampsia; pregnancy diabetes; very large baby, Diabetes test, consultation with dietician, possible late ultrasound to assess fetal size, Cesarean section	
Underweight: Less than 100 lbs. or 90% of ideal body weight	Small-for-dates baby	Attend to diet. 2nd scan at 32 weeks. Serial ultrasound to assess fetal size
Height less than 1.5 m (5 ft.)	Baby's head too big to pass through pelvis and vagina without birth trauma	Assess pelvis at 36 weeks. Consider Cesarean

Significant heart murmur	Heart disease in mother with no previous symptoms, risk of cardiac (heart) infection during labor	Appointment with heart specialist and especially so if: woman has history of rheumatic fever, symptoms of heart disease, known heart disease, or if the murmur is not due simply to the extra blood-being pumped around the body as a consequence of pregnancy. Check hemoglobin level. Possibly receive antibiotics at delivery
Uterus either large or small in relation to EDC	Multiple pregnancy, wrong dates, missed abortion, excess amniotic fluid	Check dates with scan at 16 weeks. Repeat if necessary at 20 weeks and thereafter to assess fetal size and growth and amniotic fluid
Other pelvic or abdominal abnormality	Pelvic or abdominal disease, such as ovarian cysts, ulcerative colitis, Crohn's disease	Further investigations with relevant specialist
Factors arising during pregnancy:		
Baby not felt moving by 22 weeks (see kick chart, *Feeling your baby move*)	Non-viable pregnancy, molar pregnancy (see Chapter 4) Wrong dates	Dates to be rechecked, ultrasound
Low blood count	Pregnancy anemia, poor nutrition	Test to be repeated, improve the diet (see Chapter 3). Folic acids, iron and vitamin B12 may also be indicated
Poor weight gain or weight loss	Retarded growth of the baby, poor nutrition	Tests of placental function, improve the diet (see Chapter 3)
Protein in urine with normal blood pressure	Urinary or vaginal infection, pre-eclampsia, chronic kidney disease, bladder infection	Repeat urine test, cervical swab if discharge present, special urine tests for kidney function, may need to see kidney specialist
Protein in urine, blood pressure raised	Pre-eclampsia	Admission to hospital
Sugar in urine or increased blood sugar	Pregnancy diabetes	Glucose tolerance test: if abnormal, special care
Bacteria in urine	Urinary infection, retarded growth of baby, premature labor	Will be treated and test redone to make sure it has cleared up

Blood pressure 140/90 or more, or significant increase over what was recorded at initial visit	Pregnancy hypertension, pre-eclampsia, kidney disease, retarded growth of baby	Kidney function to be checked (more urine tests). Possible admission to hospital
Significant antibodies (e.g. rhesus)	Blood disorder of baby	Will see specialist and may attend perinatal center, possible amniocentesis (see Chapter 7)
Uterus large for dates	Wrong dates, large baby, multiple pregnancy, fibroids, diabetes, excess amniotic fluid	Dates to be rechecked, repeat ultrasound scan, check for pregnancy diabetes (see Chapter 5)
Uterus small for dates or uterus not rising as in normal development	Wrong dates, retarded growth of baby, excess amniotic fluid	Check dates, program of tests to determine well-being of fetus, may include ultrasound assessment of fetal size, breathing and movement pattern, umbilical artery, flow studies, amniotic fluid volume
Too much amniotic fluid	No particular reason, no particular effect. Premature labor, malpresentation of baby, fetal abnormality, multiple pregnancy, pregnancy diabetes	Scan to assess for abnormalities and relate baby's size and growth to EDC, glucose tolerance test, possible hospital admission
Baby in wrong direction at 34 weeks (see types of presentation in Chapter 10)	Problems in labor, placenta previa (see Chapter 10)	Careful assessment of size and position by specialist, possible Cesarean section, possible vaginal delivery with team experienced in vaginal breech delivery, possible external version (turning)
Baby's head not engaged at 38 weeks in first pregnancy	Baby's head too big for pelvis; placenta in wrong place, forming obstruction, difficult presentation (occipitoposterior, see Chapter 10)	Ultrasound scan, see consultant, possible Cesarean

Vaginal bleeding before 24 weeks	Threatened miscarriage, disease or infection of cervix	Immediate ultrasound, Rhesus-negative women will have Rh immune globulin injections as bleeding can be caused in those women by baby's positive blood cells being destroyed by mother's antibodies (see Chapter 5), cervical smear.
Vaginal bleeding after 24 weeks (antepartum hemorrhage)	Placenta previa or abruption of placenta, preterm labor	Hospital admission is often recommended and is always advisable if advanced beyond 24th week. Drugs called tocolytics (labor stopping agents) may be used to quiet uterine contractions
Vaginal infection (especially herpes)	Baby may be infected if born vaginally, premature labor	Cervical swab, if herpes suspected, swab will be taken again at 36 weeks. Possibility of Cesarean delivery to avoid baby's contact with virus. Severe bacterial or monilial (yeast) infections may be treated with oral agents or vaginal creams

DANGER SIGNS

There are a number of common discomforts and irritations in pregnancy, which you may wish to check with your doctor. Some symptoms, however, indicate that there may be something seriously wrong.

You should call your doctor if you notice any of these symptoms:

1. Vaginal bleeding, unless it is merely spotting
2. Severe abdominal pain, especially if you are also bleeding vaginally
3. Continuous and severe headache, with or without blurred vision and with or without swelling of the hands and ankles
4. Excessive vomiting in which you cannot keep down any food or liquid, even water
5. Breaking of the water bag (amniotic fluid)
6. No fetal movements for 12 hours
7. A temperature of 101°F

8. Sudden swelling of the hands and ankles. If you also have blurred vision and/or severe headache as well as the swelling, you should call an ambulance (see 3, above) and/or proceed directly to hospital
9. Urinating not only frequently (which is normal in pregnancy) but with pain, signifying an infection

In cases of heavy bleeding or severe pain, you should proceed directly to the nearest hospital with a maternity unit. Pregnant women should always know of the best hospital available to their home and workplace, and, if traveling, be aware of the best source of emergency care in the immediate area.

If you are in any doubt about any symptoms during your pregnancy, do not hesitate to telephone your doctor. Remember that not only may there be some serious symptom in pregnancy, which requires prompt investigation, but you can also be ill while you are pregnant. Pregnancy does not provide immunity to other illnesses. A raised temperature, therefore, may signify an infection—which could harm you and the baby, but may not be related to the pregnancy. In the same way, appendicitis and gallstones, for example, can occur during pregnancy. If you have any worries, therefore, do consult your doctor.

WHAT YOU CAN DO YOURSELF

Prenatal care is essentially a monitoring and screening program supported by the appropriate treatment where necessary. Some of the problems of pregnancy, such as iron deficiency, for example, are conditions that you can help to prevent.

If you look back to Chapter 3: The Best of Health, you will see how much you can do to help ensure the health of the baby and yourself. A good diet, regular exercise and plenty of rest and sleep are all essential parts of prenatal care. Hospital prenatal care can do a lot, but there are some things only you can do. Regular exercises to help you control your breathing and to tone up your muscles are an important part of prenatal care. Take care to avoid those things that will positively harm your baby, such as smoking, drinking too much and using many drugs (both legal and illegal)— all described in Chapter 3.

FEELING YOUR BABY MOVE: HOW TO KEEP A KICK CHART RECORDING YOUR BABY'S MOVEMENTS

Feeling your baby kick is a good sign that it is healthy and well. You may be able to feel the baby moving by the 20th week. Knowing that the baby is moving is not only reassuring but an important part of prenatal care, so it helps both you and your doctor or midwife if you record the baby's movements, together with the time of day, on a kick chart. The hospital may provide you with a kick chart, though perhaps not until the 26th week. If not, draw one up for yourself, as shown on the opposite page.

Mark the chart according to the half-hour period in which you felt the baby move. For example, the chart is marked here for movements felt on Saturday, the last day of week 19, at ten past nine, quarter to eleven, twenty-five past twelve, half past two, ten past four, twenty to seven, twenty past eight, nine o'clock, twenty past nine, twenty to ten and eleven o'clock.

If the total number of movements in any one day is less than 10, you should record the total for that day on the chart. You should consult your doctor immediately, no matter what time of day it is, if you have not noticed any movements by the 22nd week of the pregnancy, or if 12 hours go by with no movements.

Start your kick chart when you wish, and continue with it right through your pregnancy until labor is established.

NEW DEVELOPMENTS

Prenatal testing for inherited conditions and testing before you attempt to become pregnant is advancing all the time. It is certain that the picture will have changed dramatically by the year 2000, with new tests being offered and existing tests refined. It is possible that those tests, such as chorionic villus sampling and amniocentesis, that carry a risk of miscarriage may be refined so that this risk is eliminated, or they may be superseded altogether by new tests.

The latest test being developed is known as magnetic resonance imaging (MRI). It can diagnose anything from heart disease to cancer and multiple sclerosis to birth defects. Its use is not confined to gynecology, and indeed could have very widespread applications if it were to fulfill its promise.

Instead of X-rays or sound waves, MRI uses large magnets. Much of the human body is composed of water and makes use of the natural physical properties of hydrogen atoms. If these are placed in a magnetic field, bombarded with radiowaves, they are transformed into a state of high energy. When the radiowaves are turned off, each atom releases its extra energy in the form of a faint radio signal. Carbon and phosphorus atoms will react in the same way as hydrogen atoms, each type emitting a different call sign. These signs can be converted by computer into a picture related to the type and strength of the sign. For example, fatty tissue containing a lot of water will look quite different on the screen from bone, which contains very little water.

MRI can be used to build up pictures of the developing baby before it is born and to identify any problems, including tumor, for example, that could be operated on directly after birth. The advan-

Figure 2. KICK CHART

	Week 32							Week 33							Week 34							Week 35						
	S	M	T	W	T	F	S	S	M	T	W	T	F	S	S	M	T	W	T	F	S	S	M	T	W	T	F	S
9.00							✓																					
9.30																												
10.00																												
10.30							✓																					
11.00																												
11.30																												
12.00							✓																					
12.30																												
1.00																												
1.30																												
2.00																												
2.30							✓																					
3.00																												
3.30																												
4.00							✓																					
4.30																												
5.00																												
5.30																												
6.00																												
6.30							✓																					
7.00																												
7.30																												
8.00							✓																					
8.30																												
9.00							✓																					
9.30							✓																					
10.00																												
10.30																												
11.00							✓																					
Total number of movements if less than 10 in any one day																												

tages of MRI in prenatal care are that X-rays are generally avoided because they damage the fetus, and no one is prepared to say that ultrasound is definitely safe and without risks. The disadvantage of MRI is that each machine has to be clad in heavy protective material and located well away from other machinery, as the MRI machine would otherwise magnetically attract everything else in the vicinity. There are also currently no guarantees that MRI does not carry any fetal risks, and there is to date not a great deal of experience with MRI in pregnancy.

One of the most important tests available for pregnant women is amniocentesis. This is important not only for the information it can give us about the developing baby but for the dilemma it can pose for the woman who discovers that there is something wrong with her baby. Amniocentesis, as you will see in the next chapter, is now generally performed at about the 16th week. It has already been carried out much earlier—at 11 weeks, 10 weeks and even 9 weeks—and in the future it may become much more common to have amniocentesis earlier. The possible benefits of this development are currently being evaluated in specialist centers. The indications, or reasons, for amniocentesis, have been broadened to include the evaluation of an abnormal AFD value or abnormal ultrasound. In addition, many inherited diseases may now be tested for with early genetic testing. You will read more about this in the next chapter (and see also p. 99).

7. Amniocentesis and AFP —Fetal Abnormality Screening Tests

It is now possible to test for the more common congenital defects in babies, and it is also possible to test for many rare genetic disorders (see page 157), usually only in high-risk individuals. All prenatal diagnostic tests depend on the sampling of either amniotic fluid or the baby's blood.

The tests and techniques include amniocentesis and alphafetoprotein test (discussed below), and chorionic villus sampling (described in chapter 5); and fetoscopy. Fetoscopy is a technique similar to amniocentesis but is as yet available only in specialized centers. The fetoscope is a very fine telescopic tube with a light and lens at the end. It allows for a visual inspection of any fetal malformation, and can also be used, with PUBS, to obtain a sample of the baby's blood while it is in the uterus. High-resolution ultrasonography (detailed ultrasound scan) can also be used to obtain a picture of the baby and thus to see structural (as opposed to biochemical or genetic) fetal abnormality, for example, hare lip, if it exists.

Amniocentesis, and the culture and analysis of the baby's cells taken from the amniotic fluid, means that it is now possible to diagnose large structural abnormalities in fetal chromosomes, whether these are transmitted by one or both of the parents, or whether they have occurred simply by chance. Down's syndrome, for example, can be a transmitted disorder or a sporadic one. The majority of Down's syndrome babies occur as a complete matter of chance, in which there is no transmissible genetic cause.

77

SCREENING TESTS PROCEDURE

You can see from the flow chart on page 79 that amniocentesis is not a routine test, and that you are very likely to have safer "noninvasive" tests before a decision can be made about whether or not amniocentesis is indicated (see Figure 3). Generally, an alphafetoprotein (AFP) test is done first. If the AFP level is low, amniocentesis may be offered. If the test shows a normal AFP level, you are unlikely to be offered amniocentesis, unless (1) you are over 35; (2) you are at particular risk (a previous Down's baby, for example; refer also to the Table of Positive Risk Factors in the previous chapter). If the AFP test shows a raised level, the test may be repeated to make sure that it is correct or a detailed ultrasound may be recommended. If the second AFP test shows a raised level, you will then have a detailed ultrasound scan. If this looks normal, a second scan may be performed with a possible view to PUBS or amniocentesis (for chromosomal analysis). If either shows abnormality, termination may be offered, depending on the degree of abnormality. If, however, the detailed ultrasound scan seems to indicate not abnormality but a small baby, growth scans will be performed in order to monitor the baby's progress. If growth retardation in the baby is suspected, Doppler blood flow studies may be conducted, at some research centers. This is not routine practice, however.

Alphafetoprotein tests on maternal blood and detailed ultrasound scans have to some extent, but by no means entirely, eclipsed the need for amniocentesis. For example, the detection of a raised AFP level followed by a detailed scan can identify a fetus with an open neural tube defect, in which the alphafetoprotein has leaked out of a defect of the spinal cord. The defect causes a severe abnormality which can be seen on the scan. An AFP estimation alone cannot, however, identify a closed neural tube defect because no AFP can escape since the spinal cord is closed. (Neural tube defects are discussed in Chapter 5.)

AMNIOCENTESIS

For women over 35 and for high-risk individuals, amniocentesis is the test that poses one of the biggest dilemmas of pregnancy. Amniocentesis can identify some of the most serious defects and handicaps in the unborn child. There is no treatment or cure for many of these disorders, and this means that if an amniocentesis test gives a worrying result, women have to make the very difficult decision about whether or not to have the pregnancy terminated. Some women who have been clear in their minds before-hand about what they would do if they underwent the test and were faced with the dilemma of a termination, felt quite differently

Figure 3.
Fetal Abnormality Screening Tests Procedure

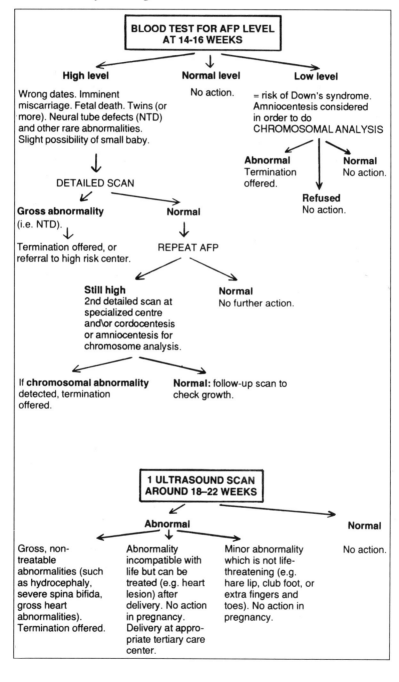

when actually confronted with the situation. Early and late termi-
nations of pregnancy are discussed in more detail later in this
chapter.

Amniocentesis, usually referred to by medical and nursing staff
as *amnio*, involves taking fluid from the amniotic cavity or amnion.
The amnion is the inner sac that surrounds the baby and the uterus.
The sac contains fluid, called amniotic fluid, which contains the
baby's urine, cells from its skin, and various chemicals produced
by the baby. One of these substances is the protein called alphafetoprotein, which is made in the baby's liver. This protein is
not usually found in non-pregnant women. Amniotic fluid can be
removed from the amnion and the cells contained in the fluid can
be analyzed and also grown in a tissue culture. The chromosomes
of these cells can then by analyzed for defects and handicap.
Alphafetoprotein levels can be tested either by testing a sample of
the mother's blood, or by testing the amniotic fluid, obtained by
amniocentesis.

What amniocentesis can reveal

In the great majority of cases amniocentesis shows that none of the
defects that the test is designed to pick up exist and that the baby
seems to be healthy.

In a very few cases, however, amniocentesis identifies one of the
following:

1. Chromosomal defects associated with congenital chro-
    mosomal abnormality and mental impairment (formerly
    termed "retardation"). Down's syndrome (which used to
    be known as mongolism) is the most common of these
    serious defects. Amniocentesis is considered to be a very
    accurate test for this type of defect.

    Amniocentesis can also test for cystic fibrosis, the most
    common genetic defect seen in the Caucasian population
    (described in Chapter 5). The test can identify 90% of
    affected fetuses but gives a 5–6% false-positive rate, and
    is therefore not offered to low-risk individuals.
2. The sex of the baby, which is important in sex-linked
    disorders such as hemophilia and muscular dystrophy
    (see Chapter 5). These diseases are usually passed on to
    male children, but women can act as carriers. Women who
    are expecting a female child have less chance of bearing a
    hemophiliac and there is a small possibility of bearing a
    child who may develop muscular dystrophy. More re-
    cently, fetal cells can in some cases be tested for certain
    types of muscular dystrophy.

    If you have the test, it is best to decide in advance if you
    would like to know the sex of the child. You can ask to be

told or you can ask not to be told. Amniocentesis and chorionic villus sampling are the only sure ways of determining the sex of the baby before birth.

3. All the inherited disorders described in Chapter 5, notably sickle cell disease, Tay-Sachs disease and thalassemia.

4. Open-neural-tube defects, such as spina bifida and anencephaly (no brain). However, amniocentesis is gradually being eclipsed for open-neural-tube defects, because an AFP blood test can pick up the greatly raised levels of alphafetoprotein characteristic of these disorders and a detailed ultrasound scan can be used to identify and visualize the handicap. (It cannot test for closed- neural-tube defects—see Chapter 5.) Some 1 to 2 in 1000 babies are found to have a neural tube defect. Half of them are miscarried and some are stillborn, or die soon after birth.

5. Amniocentesis has been offered to rhesus-negative women with antibodies (as identified by the mother's blood test at the booking visit or subsequent visit). This leads to complications caused by the mother's antibodies destroying the baby's blood cells.

    Percutaneous umbilical blood sampling has now superseded amniocentesis for this purpose so that the baby's blood is tested, rather than just the amniotic fluid. PUBS is preferable in that the baby's blood group and blood count can also be done. It can also be used as a therapeutic, as well as a diagnostic, technique: if the baby is ailing because of a rhesus incompatibility with its mother, it can be transfused while remaining in the uterus. In earlier days, such babies would have been delivered early, even prematurely. (See *Rhesus factor* in Chapter 5.)

    Any rhesus-negative woman who has amniocentesis must be given Rh immune globulin injections after the test in order to prevent the problems that would be caused by leakage of the baby's blood cells into her bloodstream (which can be caused by amniocentesis).

6. You may have heard of amniotic fluid being obtained late in pregnancy to determine the maturity of the baby's lungs. Because of much improved and highly sophisticated intensive care equipment and special drugs which can be given to the baby to activate artificially the maturity of its lungs, fetal lung maturity is less critical to fetal survival. This applies in cases of small-for-dates babies or any baby that needs to be delivered early for whatever reason. A small baby may not be developing as well as it should be in the uterus and may need to be delivered before it reaches term, the 40th week, in order to receive special care. If there is something wrong with the baby, it

may be better to deliver it, although lung maturity remains an important consideration.

7. Amniocentesis is sometimes used as a treatment, or therapeutic technique, rather than as a means of diagnosis, as we saw in PUBS in (5) above. In polyhydramnios, for example, in which there is too much liquid in the amniotic sac, some of the liquid can be drained off to relieve the pressure upon the baby. The fluid can then be tested for the conditions described above if required. This type of therapeutic amniocentesis may be done in twin pregnancies in order to relieve pressure within the mother's body and reduce the risk of premature labor.

ALPHAFETOPROTEIN BLOOD TEST

Before continuing our discussion of amniocentesis, it is well worth looking at the alphafetoprotein test. This is a simple, safe and reliable test, performed by taking a blood sample from the mother's arm. It is therefore noninvasive and without risk. It is best performed between weeks 16 and 18, but it can be performed between weeks 15 and 22.

Alphafetoprotein is a protein made by the baby's liver, and is therefore present in the amniotic fluid surrounding the baby in the uterus. It crosses the placenta, thus entering the mother's bloodstream. It is not usually found in non-pregnant women. The test measures the level of the protein. As we have seen, if it is high, it could mean that the baby has a neural tube defect (the high level being caused by the protein leaking out of the baby's spinal cord) or other rare abnormality. If it is low, it could indicate a Down's syndrome baby.

If the test produces a worrying result, it may be repeated to check the result. As the baby grows bigger, it produces more AFP. Hence, a raised AFP level may just mean that the pregnancy is more advanced than it was realized (wrong dates, in other words). It could also mean that twins (or more) are expected, which would result in higher than normal AFP levels. (See also diagram p. 79.)

For these reasons, if the second test also provides a worrying result, a detailed ultrasound scan may be recommended. This would confirm the stage of the pregnancy and therefore the baby's age and would also show whether or not the pregnancy was in fact twins or multiple. It would also identify any gross handicap and the general condition of the baby (ultrasound is described in Chapter 5).

If the ultrasound picture shows up a problem which may be part of a syndrome of defects, then a chromosomal test (PUBS or amniocentesis) may be carried out. Amniocentesis is carried out only if a chromosomal defect is suspected from the ultrasound picture;

it will not be carried out for growth retardation in the baby, wrong dates, or twins, for example.

Women who show a raised AFP level may have a higher risk of miscarriage before they undergo amniocentesis compared with those women with normal AFP levels—but this may be a reflection of the cause of the raised AFP level in the first place. In other words, if there is something seriously wrong with the baby, it may be more likely to miscarry.

Finally, in those units where good scanning facilities are available, it is easier, quicker and safer to diagnose neural tube defects by AFP and scan than by amniocentesis.

WHO IS OFFERED AMNIOCENTESIS?

Amniocentesis is not a routine test and will not be offered to every pregnant woman. It is unlikely to be offered to anyone under the age of 35, unless they are at particular risk of bearing a child afflicted with one of the disorders noted on pp. 80–81 or have been in contact with the rubella virus in the first three months of pregnancy. It may be offered to women over the age of 35 as a matter of routine and it will almost certainly be offered to those over 40 as routine practice. The reason for this is that babies with Down's syndrome are more commonly born to women over 35 or 36 and particularly over 40. The incidence rises quite sharply with age:

Amniocentesis will probably be offered to anyone whose other prenatal test results (see Chapters 5 and 6), particularly the AFP result, appear to indicate that something may be wrong with the baby. It may also be offered if one or both parents are known to be carriers of an inherited disease or if someone else in the family has such a disease—such as cystic fibrosis, Huntington's Chorea or thalassemia. If you know of the existence in your family of any of the inherited diseases described in Chapter 5, and you wish to have amniocentesis, you should ask to have it.

Having amniocentesis

Amniocentesis is safer if it is carried out using ultrasound to locate the amniotic sac, the placenta and the baby. It is best not to have it without ultrasound, as this increases the risk of miscarriage; in addition, the test may fail if insufficient liquid is obtained. After an ultrasound has been used to locate the placenta and the fetus, a "pocket" of amniotic fluid will be identified. A local anesthetic may be applied to your abdomen and a fine needle is then inserted through it. Ultrasound is used to locate the best pool of liquid in the amniotic sac and to make sure that the needle does not pierce either the placenta or the baby.

The needle then withdraws some of the amniotic fluid in much the same way that a needle withdraws blood from your arm for a blood test. The amniotic fluid is then analyzed in a number of

Table 7.1	ESTIMATED INCIDENCE OF CHROMOSOME ABNORMALITIES		
	LIVEBORN INFANTS		
Maternal Age	Down's Syndrome		All Chromosome Abnormalities
	%		%
21	1/1,500	(0.07)	1/500	(0.20)
27	1/1000	(0.10)	1/450	(0.22)
33	1/600	(0.17)	1/300	(0.33)
34	1/450	(0.22)	1/250	(0.40)
35	1/400	(0.25)	1/200	(0.50)
36	1/300	(0.33)	1/150	(0.66)
37	1/220	(0.45)	1/125	(0.80)
38	1/175	(0.57)	1/100	(1.00)
39	1/140	(0.71)	1/80	(1.25)
40	1/100	(1.00)	1/60	(1.66)
41	1/80	(1.25)	1/50	(2.00)
42	1/60	(1.67)	1/40	(2.50)
43	1/50	(2.00)	1/30	(3.33)
44	1/40	(2.50)	1/25	(4.00)
45	1/30	(3.33)	1/20	(5.00)
46	1/25	(4.00)	1/15	(6.66)
47	1/20	(5.00)	1/10	(10.00)
48	1/15	(6.70)	1/9	(11.11)
49	1/10	(10.00)	1/7	(14.28)

Source: Adapted from Hook EB, Cross PK: Interpretation of recent data pertinent to genetic counseling for Down syndrome, in Willey AM, Carter TP, Kelly S, et al (eds): *Clinical Genetics: Problems in Diagnosis and Counseling*, New York, Academic Press, 1982.

Schreinmachers DM, Cross PK, and Hook EB: Rates of trisomies 21, 18, 13 and other chromosome abnormalities in about 20,000 prenatal studies compared with estimated rates in live births, *Human Genet* 61:318, 1982.

different ways: the cells are allowed to grow and their chromosomes subsequently analyzed; an AFP measurement will also be done to determine whether or not the level is raised.

Amniocentesis is normally performed at about 16 weeks, although it can be carried out at 15 weeks or earlier and it can be done up to a few weeks later. If it is performed much earlier than 16 weeks, only small samples of fluid can be taken, there are fewer viable cells for culturing and those cells can take longer to grow and therefore longer to analyze and provide results. AFP-analysis results from amniocentesis are available within a couple of days, but the chromosomal results of an amniocentesis normally take nearly four weeks, as it takes some time to culture the cells.

Is amniocentesis safe?

Amniocentesis is not entirely safe, but it is safer if it is carried out by a doctor experienced in the technique and with the benefit of an ultrasound picture with which to guide the needle. The risk of miscarriage is somewhat less than one in a hundred. The rate at some hospitals is lower and at some it is higher. If you are considering having amniocentesis, ask your doctor: (1) if ultrasound is to be used; (2) who is going to do it; (3) what their rates of miscarriage are.

The risk-benefit ratio must be carefully considered before undergoing amniocentesis. It was noted in Chapter 2 that a 20-year-old woman has a 1 in 2,000 chance of bearing a Down's child and a 1 in 200 chance of miscarriage as a direct result of amniocentesis. The 40-year-old woman, on the other hand, has the same chance of avoidable miscarriage, of 1 in 200, but she has a greatly increased chance of having a Down's child: 1 in 100. She is therefore twice as likely to have a Down's child as she is to miscarry through having amniocentesis. The 20-year-old woman, however, is 10 times more likely to suffer a miscarriage through having amniocentesis than she is to bear a Down's child. The risks attached to amniocentesis must be carefully weighed, therefore, against the benefits it can offer to certain at-risk women.

Deciding whether or not to have amniocentesis
Amniocentesis is most likely to offer the peace of mind necessary to enjoy the rest of the pregnancy and the birth of a healthy child. It also provides valuable information for medical and nursing staff, so that they are more likely to know what, if any, abnormalities they are dealing with.

The difficulties surrounding the decision to have amniocentesis are twofold: It can cause miscarriage and the unnecessary loss of a healthy baby; or it can lead to a further dilemma, that of making a decision about whether or not to terminate the pregnancy. The safety of the technique has been described. Remember to ask your doctor the right questions to help you come to a decision.

WHAT ARE THE ALTERNATIVES?

We have seen the alternatives offered by AFP testing and detailed scans for certain disorders. There is, however, no alternative to amniocentesis for the identification of a chromosomal defect. If the woman has not presented herself until the 18th or 19th week, she may have PUBS, instead of amniocentesis, as it would by then be too late to act on the latter. PUBS is described in Chapter 5. Some experts say that the risk of miscarriage with this procedure is comparable to that of amniocentesis. Others maintain that the risk is lower or higher. In either case, you should ask your doctor: (1) if ultrasound is used with the technique; (2) who is going to do it; (3) what their rate of miscarriage is.

If you decide against these tests, and await the outcome—the wait-and-see technique—bear in mind that the majority of pregnancies result in the successful delivery of a healthy baby. However, it may be medically desirable to resolve the possibility of a problem once a risk factor has been identified, as in a worrying AFP result.

Serious problems can be identified to some degree by an AFP blood test and a detailed scan, and it may be that your doctor is already fairly certain of the nature of the problem before it is confirmed by amniocentesis. You will in any case have a talk with the physician before amniocentesis is carried out. Do raise your questions about the test, and the reasons for it in your particular case, during this talk. If for some reason your doctor does not discuss it with you, make sure that you ask for an appointment to do so.

DECIDING WHETHER OR NOT TO TERMINATE A PREGNANCY

Amniocentesis sometimes, but not in the majority of cases, reveals that there is something so wrong with the baby that a termination of pregnancy is offered. Amniocentesis reveals in only 3% of cases that there is something wrong, however; nearly half of this 3% are Down's syndrome cases. Deciding whether or not to terminate a pregnancy is clearly an extremely hard decision to make. Those who hold profound religious or humanitarian beliefs that abortion is a sin and a gross assault on the fetus would probably, in 9 cases out of 10, decide against termination. Amniocentesis has little to offer people with such strong convictions: Since the test can cause miscarriage, it may be better for them not to take the test at all.

Termination poses a dilemma, therefore, for those who are not sure whether or not to terminate the pregnancy. It may also be a very difficult choice even for those who know that they could not cope with a handicapped child or believe it wrong to bring into the world a child likely to develop an incurable, untreatable, hereditary disease.

Very occasionally, there is no alternative but to terminate the pregnancy, principally on the grounds of the mother's physical or emotional health.

The arguments against termination

Amniocentesis cannot always predict precisely the degree of handicap with these defects. It can show gross handicap incompatible with life, serious handicap that can be operated on, handicap which can be assessed while the degree of malfunction cannot, and minor handicap.

Some abnormalities, such as a structural abnormality of the heart, for example, can be operated upon shortly after delivery, resulting in a perfectly healthy child.

Remaining factors to take into account concerning the question of terminating a pregnancy include: the moral issue of loss of life (some people consider that the fetus has moral rights, too), religious beliefs, and the trauma of a late termination for both parents. In some cases, depending on the age of the mother, or other circumstances, this may be the woman's last chance to have a child. Not all people seek the perfect baby or no baby at all—some people know that they will love and care for their child regardless of whether or not it is perfect, either mentally or physically.

The arguments favoring termination

These include the question of the mother's physical and mental well-being: If the child is severely handicapped, so much so that it will die in the uterus or shortly after birth, the mother may be saved some suffering by electing for an abortion. The father and the rest of the family—particularly any other children—also need to be considered. A severely handicapped child can exert a profound influence upon its family. It will need full-time care and it may strain the emotional, physical and financial resources of the family to an unacceptable degree. The child may undergo needless suffering and die either in childhood or in early adulthood. Both parents may consider it better to forego this pregnancy and, in a year or two, seek pre-pregnancy testing from a genetic counseling service before trying again.

What happens when a pregnancy is terminated

The distinction must first be made between early and late abortions. Early abortion is performed before the end of the 13th week; after that, the term "late abortion" is used. Doctors consider early abortion more desirable than late abortion because it is a simpler and quicker operation, and because it minimizes the risks to the woman's physical and mental health. This, too, cannot be carried out after amniocentesis, as it would be too late.

Early abortion   Because this must be carried out before the end of the 13th week of pregnancy, it can be done as a consequence of chorionic villus sampling (in the 8th–10th week), or for medical or emotional reasons. It should not be done after amniocentesis, as the latter cannot be performed before the 15th week of pregnancy. The operation may be performed under a local or a general anesthetic and takes some ten minutes to remove the fetus by dilating the cervix and extracting the fetus by means of suction. Abortion at this stage of pregnancy is normally safe and simple, provided that it is carried out by appropriately trained, experienced medical staff in sterile conditions.

Dilation and evacuation—midtrimester   Between the 13th and 16th week, some centers offer a dilation and evacuation procedure which is similar procedurally to an early abortion. In highly skilled hands, this is a safer procedure than labor induction (described below). However, it is riskier than an early abortion, and women choosing this procedure need to be certain they are at a center with experience in late pregnancy termination. This, too, cannot be carried out after amniocentesis, as it would be too late.

Late abortion   This is defined as abortion from the 13th week of pregnancy onwards and is the type of termination available to those women who require an abortion after amniocentesis. The neck of the uterus, the cervix, has to be stretched so that the fetus can be removed together with the developing placenta. This can be done as in the early weeks of pregnancy, with care, without causing permanent damage to the surrounding tissues. As the pregnancy becomes more advanced, however, it is neither easy, nor medically desirable, to stretch the cervix to the required degree. If the cervix were to be stretched to that degree, it could be damaged; it could lose its elasticity and it could result in an incompetent cervix, which would lead to complications in subsequent pregnancies. Because of this, many doctors prefer to use the technique in which the natural process of birth is imitated.

The cervix dilates naturally, during labor and birth, in response to hormones, known as prostaglandins, released into the body at this time. In a late abortion, therefore, the woman is given synthetic prostaglandin in the form of a vaginal gel or suppository, or in the form of an infusion directly into the uterus, at regular intervals, until the uterine contractions that will expel the fetus, as in birth, are triggered off, causing the cervix to dilate naturally. This process is known as prostaglandin induction. If the pregnancy is being terminated because of fetal abnormality, often after 20 weeks, an irritant substance may be injected directly into the amniotic sac around the fetus.

It may be some hours before the fetus is expelled, just as it is during labor and birth. A dilatation and curettage (D & C), in which the contents of the uterus are evacuated, may be given to ensure that no fetal material, nor part of the placenta, remains. In a few cases, dilatation and curettage is offered up to the legal pregnancy termination of 24 weeks, although it is not clear at present whether D & E or prostaglandin labor induction is safer beyond 16 weeks.

Is termination of pregnancy safe?
There are risks attached to terminating a pregnancy, and these risks are higher the later the abortion. The risks include: infection, in about 3.6% of cases; prolonged bleeding in 4%; abnormal blood clotting in 0.5%; operative trauma in less than 1%; and feelings of

regret. Operative trauma, in fewer than 1 in 100 women, includes something going wrong with the anesthetic; the risk of sterility in response to the Fallopian tubes becoming blocked or by a mechanism in which the menstrual cycle is disturbed; tissue damage leading to sterility; ruptured uterus as a consequence of the powerful contractions induced by synthetic prostaglandin in late abortion; and perforation of the uterus by one of the instruments used to perform the suction or vacuum technique. However, the risks are less than the risks to the mother of carrying the pregnancy to term.

Again, the risk-benefit ratio must be carefully weighed before electing for an abortion. If the baby is severely abnormal, an abortion may be strongly recommended; if, on the other hand, amniocentesis identifies a less than severe handicap, or an operable deformity, many doctors will support those women who decide to continue with their pregnancy. Lastly, no one will compel or force you to have an abortion: This, like having amniocentesis, is a choice that only you, finally, can make, having gathered as much information as is available.

PART THREE

Weeks 29–40, the last three months

8. Childbirth Preparation Classes

Pregnant women receive prenatal care at a prenatal clinic or doctor's office, as we have discussed in Chapters 5 and 6. Women can also go to prenatal classes. These are distinct from your general prenatal care: The classes are designed to teach you about the practical and emotional aspects of pregnancy and labor, while your prenatal care concentrates on the medical aspects. Prenatal classes are known by various names such as "parenting" classes or "childbirth preparation" classes.

You will be able to go to childbirth preparation classes once a week from about the 30th or 32nd week of your pregnancy, just two months away from the estimated delivery date of your baby. The classes are valuable in that you have the opportunity to ask all the questions that you'd like to ask during your visits to the doctor but feel there isn't time for. The classes pull together all the information you have received about pregnancy and labor, answer your questions about the tests and technology of pregnancy and labor, and show you the equipment you are likely to encounter during a hospital labor.

Childbirth preparation classes vary from place to place, but, ideally, the following topics will be covered:

1. Prenatal care and hygiene. This includes many of the topics covered in Chapter 3: the importance of fresh air and exercise in pregnancy; what sort of exercises to do and how to do them; the importance of not smoking; the need for rest, sleep and relaxation; posture; back problems; diet; maternity clothing; care of the teeth; bathing. The emotional aspects of your relationship with your partner and the question of sex during pregnancy are usually dis-

cussed. (Partners are usually encouraged to attend childbirth preparation classes, and there will be a number of
talks especially for them about pregnancy, the birth and
the emotional and practical aspects of fatherhood.)
2. How the baby grows—developmental milestones of the
baby, as it is growing inside you.
3. Knowing what to expect in your own body as the weeks
go by. Coping with the common discomforts of pregnancy, including various aches and pains, backache,
minor bleeding, breathlessness, constipation, cramp,
fainting, flatulence, hemorrhoids, headaches, heart-
burn, insomnia, morning sickness, nosebleeds, pigment
blotches around the nipples and below the navel,
rashes, stretch marks, sweating, swelling of ankles, feet
and hands, tiredness, frequent urination, vaginal discharge, and varicose veins.
4. Labor and its three stages. What happens during labor.
How to recognize the early signs of labor. Breathing
exercises. Pain relief during labor. Induction. Cesareans.
5. Feeding—breast or bottle? The pros and cons. Care of the
nipples in breast-feeding and other associated problems.
What sort of bra and outer clothes to wear.
6. What you will need for the baby—clothing and equipment. How to change diapers. General care of the baby.
7. How to bathe the baby.
8. A visit to the maternity ward and labor ward. Introduc-
tion to the technology of birth. Terms explained and a look
at the fetal monitoring equipment.
9. Contraception after delivery, because you can become
pregnant quite quickly after the arrival of your baby. It is
best to delay this, however, for several months after the
birth so that you give birth to a subsequent child at a time
when you are physically and emotionally equipped to
handle another pregnancy and another baby.

Topic 1, concerning your own health, is mostly covered in Chapter 3 of this book. Topics 2 and 3 concerning the healthy development of the baby, and your medical problems, is monitored at your
prenatal clinic, as described in Chapters 5 and 6. Topic 4 is covered
in Chapter 10 and 11. The question of breast versus bottle, topic 5,
is discussed in this chapter. Topics 6 and 7 are low-tech matters and
are not, therefore, within the scope of this book. Topic 8, the use of
technology during labor and birth, is described in Chapter 11.
Contraception, topic 9, is not discussed in this book, but its importance should not be overlooked. It is certainly possible to become
pregnant surprisingly soon after the birth of a baby, but this is not
the best thing either for your body or for the first child: Very young

children need a lot of attention, so it's best to give your first at least a year or two before introducing a younger sister or brother.

BREAST OR BOTTLE?

The decision to breast- or bottle-feed, which will no doubt be discussed in detail during your class, is not so much a high-tech aspect of pregnancy and birth as an example of what can go wrong with scientific advances. Decades ago, bottle-feeding was considered to be a superior choice because of its convenience. It is now known, however, that breast-feeding supplies the baby with special nutrients and develops its immune system, among numerous other advantages. Bottle-feeding has few advantages, other than convenience. The medical evidence is now substantially in favor of

Table 8.1 BREAST-FEEDING VS. BOTTLE-FEEDING

Advantages of breast-feeding	Advantages of bottle-feeding
• Breast milk is the perfect baby food.	• Anyone can feed the baby as well as you, allowing extended family to share in feeding.
• Breast milk gives the baby protection from germs, disease and allergy, such as eczema and asthma. Breast-fed babies have fewer serious or overwhelming infections, especially diarrhea and other digestive problems, and tend to be less colicky.	• Less likely to get breast infections. • Maternal medications may be passed in breast milk and be harmful to the baby.
• Encourage baby's facial development and development of jaw and may be responsible for lower incidence of dental problems later in the baby's life.	• Certain infections such as HIV (AIDS) virus infection may be passed in breast milk.
• Encourages bonding between mother and baby.	• Seriously ill or overtired mothers may find the physical drain of breast-feeding too stressful.
• Baby will smell sweeter.	• Some women do not produce sufficient milk, leading to poor infant growth.
• Baby is less likely to become fat.	
• You do not have to bother with testing the temperature of the milk.	
• Helps you to regain your figure: Breast-feeding causes the release of a hormone, known as oxytocin, which helps the uterus to shrink back to its pre-pregnant size. Breast-feeding also uses extra calories and may help the mother burn off extra body fat gained during pregnancy.	
• Breast cancer in your later years is less likely.	
• It's more convenient—you've always got it with you.	
• It's cheaper.	

breast-feeding for those women who find they can do it. Doctors are now much more likely to offer support and guidance to the woman who encounters problems with breast-feeding than would have been the case 10 or 20 years ago.

The advantages of breast-feeding and bottle-feeding are summarized in the table on the previous page.

Physicians all over the world, and particularly pediatricians, now recognize that breast is best and encourage the mother to breast-feed if she can. However, help and support and advice about how to do it are not always so easily available. *Do* ask, right away, if you have problems with breast-feeding. If you decide to put off asking for help when you need it, you may be faced with this kind of vicious circle: You find breast-feeding your baby difficult and painful; your baby is frustrated by receiving insufficient milk, and that only with a lot of effort; this makes you feel guilty and worried, which, in turn, makes you tense and unable to relax properly while you feed the baby.

Technique is all-important in breast-feeding—and it doesn't always come naturally. Many women have had problems with feeding their babies—so don't hesitate to ask for advice at the hospital, or from your midwife, doctor, or a lactation consultant. They will give you the help you and your baby need and they will also be able to tell you about things such as breast shields, which may be beneficial. They should be able to refer you to a breast-feeding self-help group within your area, who will help you to learn the technique. Lastly, the subject of breast-feeding is covered sympathetically and systematically in the book *The Womanly Art of Breast Feeding* by La Leche League.

COMBINING BREAST AND BOTTLE

Many women, in particular women who plan to return to work shortly after delivery, may hesitate to breast-feed because they feel it will be incompatible with work. However, a variety of techniques can be used to either store pumped breast milk or to combine breast- and formula-feedings. Women who wish to combine breast- and bottle-feeding may get the best of both worlds, but may need to consult with friends, medical professionals or a lactation consultant knowledgeable about breast-feeding for working mothers.

You will learn about breast-feeding, and its advantages over bottle-feeding, in your childbirth preparation classes. Learning about something in theory, however, is never the same as doing it, so don't be disheartened if it isn't all plain sailing at first. Childbirth preparation classes are, nevertheless, helpful and practical, and particularly worth going to if this is your first child.

9. How's the Baby?

The techniques used for monitoring your baby's health while it is still growing inside you means that most fetal abnormalities can be identified at an early stage, as described in Chapters 5–7. Using them in later pregnancy, in the last 10 weeks before the expected delivery, affords doctors the opportunity of assessing the baby's well-being better than ever before and giving good prenatal care. Prenatal care is one of the most useful types of preventative medicine. This preventative health care means that the chances of a successful delivery of a healthy baby are greatly increased.

In this period, some two months before delivery, your baby will gain weight rapidly. Between weeks 33 and 40, your estimated delivery date, the baby gains more than half of what it will weigh at birth. If a baby is growing well, it is probably thriving. Monitoring the baby's health during this period consists of checking that the heart is beating normally and well, and making sure that the baby is growing well and moving.

ROUTINE TESTS

It is important at this stage to distinguish between straightforward "routine" pregnancies and those that are not. Routine tests in the last 8 to 10 weeks of pregnancy include weighing you, urine tests, measuring your blood pressure, checking your blood count and, possibly checking for diabetes, and checking the baby's size and heart beat. There will be nothing more than that provided nothing untoward is noted.

Do bear in mind that most pregnancies are straightforward and they therefore do not demand the entire array of medical technology—it is there for those who need it.

SEQUENCE OF EVENTS

What normally happens in these last two months of pregnancy is that you visit the prenatal clinic once every two weeks and then, in the last month of pregnancy, once a week. You will have the routine tests described above. You and the baby will be assessed for labor as described in this chapter: How well will the baby stand up to the rigors of labor and delivery; is it in the right position for a vaginal delivery; and will it get through? (This last question requires an assessment of the size of its head and the size of your pelvis, in order to eliminate the possibility of cephalo-pelvic disproportion.) The baby's general well-being is assessed, as is its heartbeat. It is important at this time for doctors to determine any problems, by a combination of scanning techniques and clinical judgment, of each individual case, so that decisions may be considered concerning induced labor and Cesarean delivery, if necessary.

HEALTHY AND KICKING

You may notice five important symptoms in your body, indicating that the baby is well and progressing normally towards delivery. These include the baby's movements, which you can record on a kick chart, as shown at the end of Chapter 6. (Be sure to tell your doctor if you have felt no kicks in any 12-hour period.)

A second symptom is breathlessness: You may feel quite short of breath even climbing stairs or walking up a small hill. This happens for two reasons: The first is that your lungs are working twice as hard as usual, in order to supply both you and the baby with oxygen, and this is made all the harder because by now the baby is so large that it is pressing up against your lungs. This breathlessness is a common symptom of the last few weeks of pregnancy; but don't worry, the baby will receive enough oxygen, even though you'll sometimes be panting with the effort.

A third symptom you'll notice is that you seem to want to urinate every five minutes—and you may be caught short now and again. This happens partly because the baby is pressing upon all your internal organs, including your bladder, and partly because your muscles become smoother and softer in tone, in preparation for the birth when they will be required to stretch to the limit. When you urinate normally, you relax your muscles; when you are pregnant these muscles tend to relax of their own accord whether you want them to or not. This is what causes the feeling that you need to urinate and, sometimes, slight incontinence.

A fourth symptom that you may have noticed are small and irregular contractions. These happen throughout pregnancy and you'll feel them as a tightening in the abdominal area. Towards the end of pregnancy, when they are known as Braxton Hicks contractions, they become more pronounced, although they are still nothing like labor contractions. At this stage they will last for no more than 20 seconds or so. When you go into labor, contractions will be more powerful and they will last for 40 seconds or more. Some experts maintain that these contractions occur throughout pregnancy in order to encourage the blood flow in the placenta, which brings oxygen to the baby.

A fifth symptom that indicates everything is progressing normally is what used to be known as "lightening," and is in fact the engagement of the baby's head in the upper part of the pelvis. (See Figure 4.) This engagement of the baby's head usually occurs after the 36th week. All the way through pregnancy your uterus expands upwards in your body in order to accommodate the baby's increasing size. At the 12th to 13th week of pregnancy the baby is still quite low down in your body but after this it steadily rises upwards until the 36th week. The lower part of the uterus expands, in preparation for the baby's birth, and the baby moves downwards a little. The baby's head engages in the upper part of the pelvis ready for delivery just a few weeks later (this pressure is one of the factors, incidentally, that makes you want to urinate a lot).

The position of the baby's head and that of your uterus is noted on each of your visits to the doctor, so that the baby's downward movement, when it comes at roughly 36 weeks, or later, may be noted in your chart as "engaged." When the doctor examines you for the position of the baby, he or she can also estimate the size of the baby and whether it is, generally, the right size for that week of pregnancy.

Kicking by the baby, your breathlessness, wanting to urinate frequently, minor contractions and engagement are all good signs that the baby is growing and everything is progressing smoothly.

THE BABY'S WELL-BEING

A baby's health used to be assessed by measuring the mother's urine or blood levels for various chemicals produced by the placenta and comparing those levels with what the levels should be. These days, however, ultrasound scans, Doppler scans and cardiotocography (fetal monitoring) are used in order to obtain much more precise information.

Ultrasound scan

The baby's heart can be seen beating by using this visual method of assessing the baby's heart and thus its well-being. In addition, if the doctor suspects that something is not quite right, you may be given an ultrasound scan to determine the baby's size, in case it is not growing properly, and to determine any abnormality, during

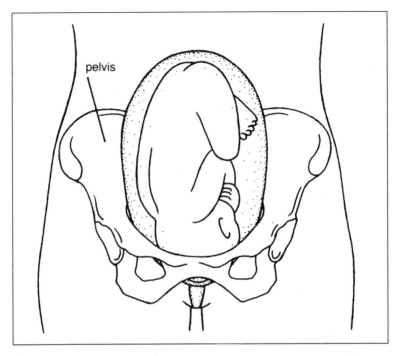

pelvis

Figure 4. *The baby often descends a few weeks before delivery so that its head engages in the upper part of the pelvis. The head may not engage until the onset of labor, however. This engagement of the baby's head is recorded on your medical record as E, eng. or engaged.*

this period of 30 weeks and onwards in the pregnancy. A Doppler scan (as described in Chapter 5) measures the blood flow, both uterine and placental, and is currently being assessed for its ability to judge the function of the placenta. If the placenta matures early, for example, it can outgrow its value and therefore no longer be capable of supplying the baby with what it needs for life. If this happens the baby has to be delivered as quickly as possible, either by inducing labor early or by Cesarean section, in order to prevent the baby's rapid deterioration.

The baby's heartbeat
If a baby is growing well, generally speaking, it probably is well. The well-being of the baby depends on an adequate supply of oxygen, which it obtains from oxygenated blood, and this is why blood flow in the placenta is assessed, with Doppler, and why the baby's heartbeat is checked in a number of possible ways. These include *looking* at the heart beating with ultrasound; *listening* to it beating with Doptone ultrasound; *listening* with a special stetho-

scope (very low-tech); or using a fetal heart monitor, known as cardiotocography or fetal monitor apparatus for a combined *auditory* and *graphic* picture.

The baby's heart beats at around 120 to 160 beats per minute, much faster than its mother's, which beats at about 70–80 per minute. The baby's heartbeat is not only much quicker than its mother's, but lighter as well. The two cannot therefore be confused.

The baby's heart is much more audible after the 28th week of pregnancy, and so a doctor can listen to it, without using any machines, with a special stethoscope shaped like a trumpet, known as a fetal stethoscope, which is placed on the mother's abdomen.

Fetal monitoring equipment allows for a much more sensitive assessment of the baby's well-being than could ever be achieved by listening with a fetal stethoscope. The machine incorporates a printout known as a cardiotocograph (CTG), and can be used both before and during labor. The tracing shown on the printout paper records the "ups and downs" of the baby's heart beat. The tracing is assessed by its rate in beats per minute, the presence or absence of accelerations or decelerations (in which the heart rate either increases or decreases for a short period), and the variation in the heart rate from beat to beat. The heart beat is normally variable, so small increases or decreases in the beat for a short time are nothing to worry about.

With either internal or external monitoring, the baby's heartbeat in response either to contractions or to its own movements are noted (the mother indicates when she feels it moving). If the baby's heartbeat speeds up a little in response, that's good; if it doesn't, a decision has to be made about whether or not the baby will be able to withstand labor; or whether it would be better to induce it, while monitoring it continuously with the fetal scalp electrode; or, finally, delivering it by Cesarean if necessary.

How well will the baby withstand labor?

Fetal heart monitoring, or cardiotocography, allows an assessment to be made of fetal heart function; in other words, how well the baby's heart is likely to stand up to labor. The strength of the baby's heart beat is recorded on the monitor, with particular reference to how well the heart copes during a contraction and how the baby's heart responds to its own movement. As well as the cardiotocogram, the baby's growth and the mother's condition are taken into account when predicting how well the baby will withstand labor.

Using the fetal heart monitor

There are two methods of monitoring the baby's heart by electronic means: the external method, in which a transducer and a belt is placed around the mother's abdomen and the baby's heartbeat picked up; and the internal method involving a fetal scalp electrode, which is used only after the water bag has broken and labor has started, or after induction (see Chapter 10). With this method the monitor is passed up through the woman's vagina, and the end-point (a probe with a clip on the end) fixed under the skin of the baby's scalp or buttocks.

Internal fetal heart monitoring is clearly a task only for skilled and experienced medical practitioners. Interpreting the data correctly is, of course, crucial in order to prevent the possibility of unnecessary surgery, in the form of a Cesarean.

The action of the baby's heart can be monitored every day, if required; or ultrasound scans can be given every two weeks.

Telemetry (described in Chapter 11) is currently being evaluated as a means of external fetal heart monitoring at home, prior to labor, and the results conveyed via computer/telephone link to the hospital. This would enable women to have external fetal heart monitoring at home instead of in the hospital.

FOR AND AGAINST FETAL HEART MONITORS

Electronic heart monitors can, ideally, be used as a part of prenatal assessment of pregnancy and fetal well-being, when it is suspected that complications may exist, and during labor. Some doctors feel that routine use of such monitors is a good thing, particularly in labor, whether or not there is any reason to suspect that the pregnancy and the eventual labor are to prove anything other than straightforward.

As it has been noted before, however, no one is able to predict with complete accuracy a straightforward pregnancy or labor: You cannot know for certain until afterwards.

It is only the external method of fetal heart monitoring that is used in the weeks before labor starts (other methods are described in Chapter 11). Briefly, advocates of the technique believe that monitoring should be a routine part of prenatal care and care during labor and delivery. Critics maintain that both external and internal monitoring give rise to a higher rate of Cesarean deliveries and inductions, when there is no need, simply because of quite normal irregularities in the baby's heartbeat. Critics also maintain that internal monitoring can damage the baby and can introduce infection both to mother and baby. There are, however, no known instances of serious damage to the baby, i.e. brain damage, although minor cuts and mild infections have been known.

"STRESS" AND "NON-STRESS" TEST

You may have read about either of these two tests, neither of which has quite the significance they used to have. The stress test was introduced many years ago in order to test fetal heart function in the presence of uterine contractions. These contractions were induced by means of the drug, Syntocinon (the synthetic version of oxytocin), in the form of an intravenous infusion. Stress testing is a useful way of assessing placental function and the baby's reaction to labor. However, stress testing is expensive, cumbersome and requires highly trained staff and has some risks. Therefore, most obstetricians try to avoid extensive stress testing. When used, it is usually performed weekly or twice weekly.

Non-stress testing (NST) involves simply monitoring the baby and observing the heart rate for speed-ups or accelerations. A "reactive" reading with good accelerations is a reliable sign of fetal well-being. However, "false-positive" readings in which a healthy baby may not appear reactive may lead to additional tests, and the NST cannot predict future adverse events. However, it is relatively inexpensive and easy to administer and is widely used in the United States for high-risk pregnancies.

The Biophysical Profile involves ultrasound assessment of fetal heartbeat, movement, breathing patterns and the placenta and amniotic fluid. It requires an experienced specialist to administer the procedure and interpret the results. Many specialists feel that a reactive NST and a normal amniotic fluid volume on ultrasound is the equivalent of a normal biophysical profile; other specialists feel that the biophysical profile is a better test of fetal well-being.

REASON TO WORRY?

Most pregnancies proceed with no serious problems. There are, however, very occasionally signs and symptoms in a pregnancy or in the mother's condition that merit investigation, and sometimes appropriate treatment. (*Signs* are what doctors observe about you, and *symptoms* are what you notice about yourself.)

The major signs and symptoms to be taken seriously include:

1. the baby's movements fading away
2. retarded growth in the baby
3. significant weight loss by the mother

Other signs and symptoms, as noted in the Table of Danger Signs in Chapter 6, include: vaginal bleeding, severe abdominal pain, continuous and severe headache, blurred vision, swelling, excessive vomiting and breaking of the waters.

ADMISSION TO THE HOSPITAL

The signs and symptoms noted above indicate that immediate hospital admission is desirable in order that the mother may have complete rest, and mother and baby be closely monitored. The cause of the problem can be identified and treated appropriately.

Swelling of the hands and ankles, for example, can be due to rising blood pressure and is also associated with pre-eclampsia, a condition that can be treated if detected in time but could prove dangerous or fatal to both mother and baby if untreated (see Chapter 5).

SMALL FOR DATES

There are various reasons for a baby being smaller than expected and not all those reasons signify that there is anything wrong. The baby may be small because you are of a small build, or—if you are Asian, for example—because this is a normal racial characteristic. The baby could be small because you have continued to smoke or to drink heavily throughout the pregnancy. The baby might simply be small because there has been a mistake in the dates; however, an ultrasound scan can identify the correct age of the baby by its size and its stage of development. Poor nutrition or chronic anemia could also be causes.

The baby could be small because of some "insult" early on in the pregnancy—for example, an infection such as rubella, or an exposure to chemicals such as nicotine, from the mother smoking, or very large amounts of alcohol.

Other conditions associated with small-for-dates babies are maternal conditions that interfere with the energy supply to the baby, such as high blood pressure, pre-eclampsia, diabetes or being underweight. It is sometimes necessary to deliver these babies early so that they can receive adequate care and nourishment in intensive care.

EARLY DELIVERY

If it is decided for any reason that the baby is not doing well, a decision may be made to deliver the baby before the estimated date of delivery. A baby can be delivered vaginally by inducing labor early, or by Cesarean (described in the next chapter) up to 3 weeks before the estimated date of delivery. The baby is then described as pre-term, rather than premature. A premature baby is one that has arrived more than three weeks before expected and one that has a somewhat increased chance of respiratory problems in its first few days, maybe necessitating special care. Drugs can be given to activate artificially the baby's lungs to speed them towards maturity but these work only if administered early in the third trimester (approximately weeks 29 to 33). The baby may also require help with breathing, in which case it can be put on a ventilator and kept very warm while it builds up its fat reserves.

Premature babies born after the 30th week of pregnancy have a 90–95% chance of survival with help from intensive care, provided that no severe fetal abnormality or rhesus incompatibility exists, which may have caused the premature labor in the first place. If the baby is born between the 35th and 37th week of pregnancy, its chance of survival is over 95%.

Intensive care is one of the best products of medical research and technology. A baby who is born prematurely may not be fully developed and may be incapable of survival without intensive care. Because its lungs have still to mature, it may have serious breathing problems, leading to respiratory failure, a common cause of death in premature babies. These problems are very often successfully resolved, however, by placing the baby on a ventilator in intensive care.

MECHANICS OF LABOR

In normal pregnancies, all you have to worry about is the routine tests noted at the start of this chapter and what are known as the mechanics of labor—in other words, will the baby get through?

A baby needs, ideally, to be in the right position to be born, and the mother's birth canal and pelvis have to be of sufficient size in relation to the baby's head for the baby to be born safely with the minimum trauma to it and to the mother.

It is suspected, very occasionally, that the baby's head is too large for the mother's pelvis—this is known as cephalo-pelvic dispro-portion (cephalo meaning head). This can happen with diabetic women (because their babies are sometimes very large with large shoulders). It can also happen in women of very short stature with very narrow pelvises.

Where cephalo-pelvic disproportion is identified, the delivery may have to be by Cesarean section in order to prevent serious injury both to the mother and baby.

THE BABY'S POSITION

As for the baby's position, an examination or ultrasound scan can establish which position the baby is in. If it is in a less than ideal position for birth, it may be turned or it may be left as it is. Turning involves a doctor manipulating the baby's head by feeling your abdomen and gently coaxing the baby around so that it assumes the desired position. If this is to be done, it will not be before the 32nd week of pregnancy in case the baby simply turns around again; and it cannot be done late in the pregnancy because the baby is by then too big to be maneuvered in this way.

A baby may present itself for birth in a number of different ways, described in the next chapter. If a baby is presenting itself shoulder first, in what is known as a transverse lie, for example, it will be impossible for it to get through the mother's pelvis unless it is turned. In such cases, if the baby cannot be turned, it is delivered by Cesarean section. If it is a breech baby (i.e. head up), it may either be turned between weeks 32 and 36; or monitored very carefully in labor when it may be born vaginally with success; or it may have to be delivered by Cesarean (all discussed more fully in the next chapter). Turning a breech baby is much more difficult than turning a transverse lie and many obstetricians now prefer not to attempt this maneuver as it may result in complications, such as the detachment of the placenta.

Many experts now believe that it is best not to turn the baby, unless it is in a transverse lie, as (1) there may be reasons why the baby has not turned itself into the normal position for birth, such as an obstruction, as in placenta previa; and (2) complications can ensue as a result of maneuvering the baby in this way. These problems are discussed more fully in the next chapter.

NO WORRIES

The great majority of pregnancies advance with no serious problems through labor to the successful delivery of a healthy baby. Your steady weight gain in these last few weeks before delivery is a good sign that everything is going well. By the time your baby arrives it is most likely that it will be perfectly developed with all the finishing touches—hair, eyebrows, eyelashes, fingernails and toenails. Remember that the vast majority of babies are healthy, so your baby has a good chance, the more so if you keep yourself in good health.

10. Preparing for Birth

In the last four weeks before your estimated date of delivery, you will probably be keenly aware of what is happening to your body, and what it means for you and for the baby. You will also be aware of how the baby is presenting her- or himself for birth from your visit to the prenatal clinic. You may also be wondering when your water bag will break; and, if any problems have presented themselves, your doctor may have talked to you about the possibilities of induction or delivery by Cesarean section. This chapter covers the 36th week of pregnancy to delivery and therefore comprises all the topics mentioned above.

WHAT YOU MAY BE FEELING

By the 36th week of pregnancy, many women start to feel that they have been pregnant for long enough and that they would like to get on with labor and see their baby. Tiredness, the cumbersome bulk of pregnancy, constipation and/or frequent urination, may all combine to make you fed up with the long weeks of pregnancy. However, these last four weeks are important for the baby's development: Its heart and lungs mature, and its fat deposits are greatly increased (which means it can survive much better once it is born). Your weight gain is partly a sign that the baby is growing at the rate that it should in this last valuable month of its protected existence.

The baby's movements, your breathlessness, wanting to urinate frequently, Braxton Hicks contractions and engagement of the baby's head are the five signs (described in detail in the previous chapter) that indicate the baby is well and progressing towards its birth. You may start to feel a sense of elation and renewed energy at the impending arrival of the baby now that there are only four weeks to go.

107

ROUTINE CHECKS IN THE LAST FOUR WEEKS

You will probably have a prenatal check once a week during the last month of pregnancy and you will also be attending your prenatal class once a week (see Chapter 8). Your routine checks will include tests for signs of hypertension and pre-eclampsia. High blood pressure, known as hypertension, is detected by repeated measurements of your blood pressure. If your blood pressure rises in late pregnancy your heart cannot pump blood around your body as efficiently as it would if it were maintained at a lower level. This means that your baby may not be receiving sufficient nourishment and oxygen—because the placenta is receiving less blood. High blood pressure may cause your baby to be a little smaller than it otherwise would have been, which means it may become distressed during labor, and it is also one of the signs, together with swelling of the ankles and hands, and protein in the urine, of pre-eclampsia. High blood pressure can be brought down and maintained at an optimum level by drugs which do no harm to the baby.

Blood pressure measurements and urine tests will be made in these last four weeks of pregnancy in order to identify any problems. Rhesus-negative women with antibodies, diabetic women and all hypertensive women, for example, will be monitored closely for complications in their pregnancy and approaching delivery. The existence of protein in the urine together with a raised blood pressure and swelling of the hands and ankles are the classic signs of pre-eclampsia, a potentially dangerous condition that, if untreated, may cause the mother to have seizures and the baby to be damaged. Such women may need to be admitted to the hospital for rest and medical observation prior to delivery.

If routine tests indicate that there is anything amiss, ultrasound scans and fetal heart monitoring may be carried out to identify any problem more precisely, and to give information about the baby's health and its chances of a successful delivery. Scans were discussed in detail in Chapter 5 and fetal heart monitoring was described in the previous chapter.

FALSE LABOR

The true early signs of labor are described in the next chapter, but it is worth noting here the reasons that women are sometimes misled into believing that they are in labor when they are not. All the way through pregnancy you may feel some very minor uterine contractions, a sense of tightening in the abdominal area. In the last few weeks of pregnancy these contractions become more pronounced and they are sometimes painful. These are known as Braxton Hicks contractions (after the man who identified them).

Although Braxton Hicks contractions occur towards the end of pregnancy and can be painful, they are irregular and they do not cause the cervix to dilate, which means you are not in labor. Your uterus may contract every 20 minutes or so for about 20 to 30 seconds, whereas the contractions felt in the first stage of labor last for 40 seconds or more, up to 1 minute.

Sometimes the first thing to happen at the start of labor is the appearance of a mucus plug from the vagina. This is known as a "show" of mucus and it is sometimes tinged with blood, giving it a pinkish appearance. This is a sign that the cervix is starting to dilate: Up until labor starts the plug remains in place, preventing infection entering the uterus. As the cervix starts to dilate in preparation for the delivery, the plug comes out. This is followed sooner or later by the water bag breaking (rupture of the membranes that surrounded the baby) described on pp. 118–119. The cervix then dilates further and further, and you will start to experience the contractions of the first stage of labor.

It may be that you don't notice the pinkish mucus plug but you will probably notice when your water bag breaks. Once the water has broken, you can safely assume that the "show" has appeared, and you should now be admitted to the hospital.

False labor, then, is characterized by irregular contractions lasting for no more than 30 seconds, no "show" and no rupture of the membranes.

However, Braxton Hicks contractions can start to seem like the real thing, particularly if it is your first baby. General anxiety, especially in women who live some distance from the hospital, who will have to call an ambulance to get them to the hospital, can seem to intensify these irregular contractions to the degree where they seem to be regular and pronounced. The woman is then quite sure that the baby has begun its descent towards the birth canal. As soon as women in false labor are admitted to the hospital, however, the contractions resume their usual irregular pattern, as well as now seeming less strong and less frequent.

If you are in any doubt at any time, you should call your doctor or the hospital or birthing center. If they advise you to come in to be examined, they will be able to tell whether or not you are in labor by looking at your cervix (the neck of the uterus). If it is not dilated, you are not in labor; if it is, your labor has begun.

The hospital is likely to suggest that you come in, so that someone can examine your cervix, because it is possible to be in the first stage of labor even if your water bag has not broken and you have not had a show. In other words, a show probably means labor, and your water bag breaking—whether there has been a show or not—also means labor. However, the absence of a show and the failure of the membranes to rupture does not necessarily mean that you are not in labor.

Clearly, it can sometimes be difficult to know if you are in labor or not—so do not hesitate to telephone the hospital if you are in any doubt at all.

If, on the other hand, there has not been any noticeable show, and your water bag has not broken, but the first stage of labor has actually passed, you may fail to appreciate that you are already in the second stage of labor. This is characterized by pronounced and painful contractions coming regularly, and gradually increasing in frequency; the contractions will last for at least 40 seconds. If this happens, you should proceed directly to the hospital. By the time you get there, you may be in a fairly advanced stage of labor. You should *on no account* attempt to drive anywhere yourself.

HOW THE BABY PRESENTS ITSELF FOR BIRTH

It was noted in the previous chapter that the baby's position, in preparation for birth, can be established from the 32nd week. If the baby is to be turned, so that it is in the best position for birth, it must be done between the 32nd week and the 36th week. It cannot be done earlier because the baby may simply turn itself around again and it cannot be done after the 36th week because the baby by then will be too large to maneuver; additionally, many obstetricians believe that this should not be done at all.

The baby's position for birth is described as its lie, its presentation and its position. (See Figures 5, 6 and 7.)

The baby's lie

The "lie" describes the way that the baby is lying in your body. It may be lying in a longitudinal lie with its head up or head down, or it may be lying across your body in a transverse lie.

Nearly all babies, before the 32nd week, change their position frequently and may be in the breech position: This is a longitudinal lie with the head up and breech or buttocks downwards. After the 32nd week, most babies turn themselves so that 96% are now in a longitudinal lie with their heads down. Some 3%, however, do not turn and remain in the breech position. The remaining 1% are made up of babies who assume an oblique lie and a transverse lie, in which the shoulder is presented for birth, in which case the baby must be delivered by Cesarean.

Babies are most safely born if they are in a longitudinal lie with their heads down. Some 4%, therefore, need special management before labor starts in order that the baby does not suffer. This means establishing before birth whether the pelvis is large enough to accommodate the baby comfortably if it is a breech presentation. If it is not large enough, a Cesarean delivery is advised. In the case of a baby in a transverse lie, the baby may be turned, as this involves only a 90 degree turn rather than the 180 degree turn that would be required by a breech.

Factors determining the choice between vaginal breech delivery and Cesarean include the size of the mother's pelvis and the size of the baby's head, location of the placenta and a number of other factors, such as raised blood pressure or diabetes.

The baby's presentation

The baby's lie determines partly how it will be born, but so partly does its presentation and position. Of the 96% of cephalic, head-down lies, 99.7% of these are what is known as vertex presentations. This means that the baby's head is well flexed with its chin on its chest, and the vertex, the crown of the head, is the part touching the cervix and to be born first. The bone at the back of the baby's head is known as the occiput and it is this that presents first when the head is well flexed to the chest.

The remaining 0.3% present their face (0.2%) or brow (0.1%) for birth, in presentations known as face presentation or brow presentation. Both involve a prolonged and difficult labor. Face presentations can be delivered vaginally provided that the chin is anterior (the back of the baby's head faces the mother's spine), but brow are always delivered by Cesarean (unless they spontaneously become face or vertex) as they cannot fit into the pelvis in order to descend.

Breech presentations have been described above. It is possible to deliver these babies vaginally safely in 30–40% of cases, but they are often delivered by Cesarean. Apart from factors such as cephalo-pelvic disproportion and fetal heart function to be taken into consideration, the reason for the breech presentation has to be taken into account. The placenta may be in such a position as to make it impossible for the baby to assume a head-down position or there may be some other obstruction, such as a fibroid. (See also *placenta previa* and *placental abruption*, later in this chapter.)

The baby's position

Most of us think in terms of the baby's lie and presentation when we think of its position. However, technically speaking, the baby's position describes which way it is facing. If the baby is facing towards your spine, it is said to be in an anterior position and labor is likely to be easier. If the baby is facing outwards, however, with the back of its head to your spine, it is said to be in a posterior position. Labor may be slower and it is also likely to produce severe backache in the mother. (The occipito-posterior position, noted in Chapter 6 in the Table of Positive Risk Factors, describes a baby who presents for birth with the back of its head well up, with the head well flexed to the chest, in a posterior position.)

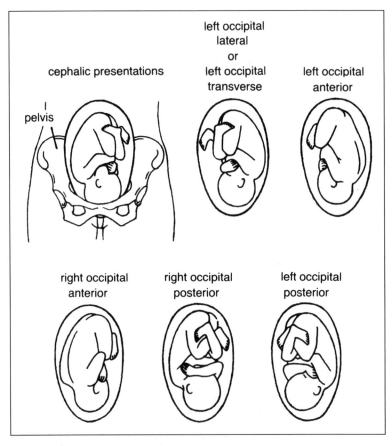

Figure 5. *Nearly 96% of babies will present for birth with well-flexed head (i.e., with the head well tucked into the chest) to the mother's pelvis as illustrated above. The position of the baby's back and occiput (the bone at the back of the baby's head) will vary, however. In the illustrations top left and top center the back and occiput directly face either the right or left side of the pelvis. In the illustrations top right and bottom left they face the front or anterior part of the pelvis, but again either towards left or right. In the last two illustrations, bottom center and bottom right, the baby's back and occiput face the posterior aspect or back of the pelvis, either right or left as with the other positions.*

The baby's lie, presentation and position

The baby's lie, then, describes the relationship between the spine of the baby and the spine of the mother. It describes the north-south axis. If the baby's spine is on a long axis to its mother's, whether head up or head down, it is said to be in a longitudinal lie; if the long axis of the baby (its spine) lies at right angles to the mother's spine, it is said to be in a transverse lie; and if it is on an oblique or

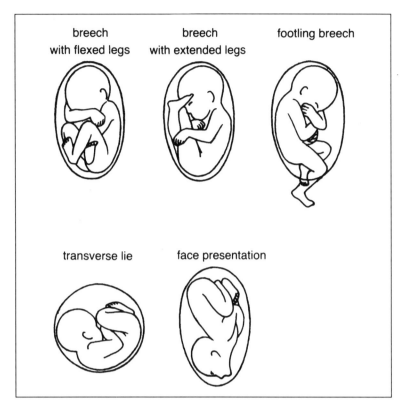

Figure 6. *96% of babies present the head at the pelvis, some 3% remain in a breech presentation and less than 1% comprise transverse and oblique lies. A breech baby with flexed legs is known as a complete breech (top left); a breech with its legs extended as a frank breech (top center); and a breech in which a foot presents first as a footling breech (top right).*

Of those who assume a transverse or oblique lie, some present their shoulder for birth in what is known as a transverse lie with its spine lying at right angles to the mother's spine (bottom left). Oblique or diagonal lies account for the rest.

Of the 96% of babies who present head down, 99.7% present with heads well flexed to the chest, 0.2% present their face (lower right) and 0.1% present their brow, both due to excessive extension of the head.

diagonal axis, the lie is described as oblique. The presentation simply describes what part of the baby is presenting itself at the pelvic brim and, therefore, which part of the baby is to be born first. The position describes which way the baby is facing.

These three coordinates are all based on the relationship of the baby's head to the mother's pelvis, both of which are three-dimensional. There are, therefore, a number of different positions that the baby can assume.

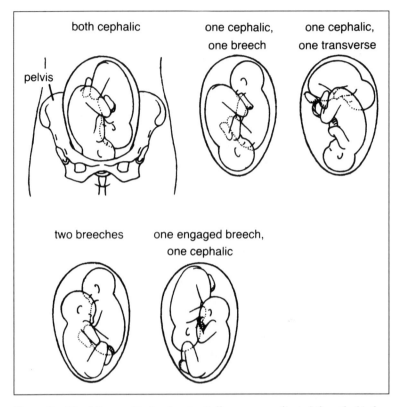

Figure 7. *The delivery of twins is potentially more complicated than the birth of a single baby, but it is possible to deliver both babies vaginally provided that no additional complications exist. These illustrations show some of the possible variations in the presentation of twins.*

YOUR MEDICAL RECORD

Your medical record will be marked with the details of the way that the baby is presenting itself for birth. Typically, prenatal records show: date, week of pregnancy, weight, urine alb. sugar (protein or sugar in the urine), BP (blood pressure) and height of fundus. (Fundus means top of the uterus. The uterus can be felt below the navel in early pregnancy. As the pregnancy advances and the baby grows bigger, the uterus expands upwards so that towards the end of the pregnancy the top of the uterus can be felt underneath the rib cage. Assessing the height is important, therefore, as this assesses the baby's growth and the development of the pregnancy.) Your records will also show the baby's presentation and position (the details of the lie, presentation and position), and relation of presenting part to brim (the position of the baby's head in relation to the brim of your pelvis, described as how many fifths of the head can be felt. When it is fully descended, when one fifth of the head can be felt, it is described as engaged. This usually happens between the 38th week and the onset of labor, although it may happen earlier.

The rest of your record will carry details of fetal heart and fetal movement. The record also records any edema (swelling), blood count (as Hb), date of next visit and any special notes (for example, that you are taking iron).

TURNING THE BABY

It was noted in the previous chapter that the baby may be turned by the doctor if it is in a head-up position or in an oblique or transverse lie, in order to avoid having to do a vaginal breech delivery or Cesarean for breech babies, and a Cesarean for oblique and transverse lies. However, this is by no means either automatically or even frequently done: Many specialists now agree that it is not a good thing to try to turn the baby. Those that intend to do it often leave it until the 34th week in case the baby decides to turn itself. You will remember that it is more difficult to do after the 36th week as by then the baby is too large to maneuver.

There are certain dangers attached to trying to turn the baby in the uterus and these include: (1) the placenta may become detached; (2) the maneuver may be quite painful for the mother; (3) it may cause premature labor; (4) in the case of rhesus-negative women, blood cells may leak from the baby into the mother's blood, thereby setting up the problems of rhesus incompatibility in which the baby's rhesus positive cells may induce the mother's rhesus-negative blood to produce antibodies. These in turn may cross the placenta into the baby and destroy its cells (see *Rhesus factor* in Chapter 5).

For all these reasons it is often decided not to try to turn the baby and, instead, to elect for a Cesarean. This is known as an elective Cesarean, in other words, a planned Cesarean, and is described later in this chapter. (Non-elective Cesarean, or emergency Cesarean, is the same operation, although unplanned, and carried out as an emergency after labor has started in response to some life-threatening complication only apparent at a late stage.)

BREECH BABIES

Most babies that are not in the ideal position for birth are breech babies, and the remaining few are oblique or transverse lies.

Hospital procedures for the delivery of breech babies vary: Some obstetricians will try to turn the baby; some will attempt a vaginal delivery; others will elect to do a Cesarean. It is possible to deliver a breech baby vaginally, but it may prove extremely difficult and hazardous. Extra care must be taken, with all the necessary specialists on hand (an anesthesiologist must be available, for example, in case an emergency Cesarean is called for.) It is not uncommon to induce a breech presentation at term, the 40th week, or if the woman has high blood pressure. A breech delivery may typically involve not only induction, but also a cut (episiotomy), forceps and an epidural (all described in the next chapter) in order to control carefully the delivery. Because of the potential problems with a vaginal breech delivery, some hospitals routinely elect for all breech babies to be delivered by Cesarean.

Types of breech presentation

The term "complete breech" describes a baby who has assumed the same attitude as a cephalic (head-down) presentation, except that it is head-up; in other words, its limbs are flexed. Incomplete breeches comprise the other types of breech, which include frank breech, footling breech and knee presentation. Frank breeches present with legs extended and footlings with the feet.

Footling breech   The chief problem with a footling breech presentation, in which the baby's feet are the part to be born first, is that the feet do not present a sufficiently strong stimulus to the cervix to cause it to dilate to allow the birth of the baby. The baby needs to be able to breathe, but if the pelvis is small, the baby's head may become stuck at the brim of the pelvis. Normally, the head comes first and pushes upon the cervix, causing it to dilate sufficiently, eventually, for the head to be born. The rest of the baby's body is then born quite quickly. When the baby presents itself feet first, the full dilatation of the cervix may take some time and it may be that the baby is so long awaiting delivery that it becomes distressed (from lack of oxygen). Because the baby's feet present an insufficiently strong stimulus to the cervix and because it may not, therefore, be fully dilated when the mother has the urge to push, the head may become stuck. Additionally, as the baby's feet do not present a snug fit to the pelvis, the umbilical cord may drop down through the cervix and go into spasm or be compressed, hampering the baby's circulation and therefore its oxygen supply. This may lead to fetal distress.

The main problem with a breech baby, whether it is a footling breech or a frank breech, is making sure that the baby's head is born relatively quickly—in other words, the second stage of labor must be quick in order to prevent the baby being asphyxiated. A breech baby can become stuck, and therefore quickly short of oxygen, in any one of three places: above the brim of the pelvis or in any part of the pelvis; in a partly dilated cervix; and on the perineum, which is why an episiotomy must be performed.

Frank breech   If the baby is in a bottom presentation with its legs up towards its neck, known as a frank breech, the baby can negotiate the birth canal in this position as the cervix readily dilates fully, usually allowing the head to follow without delay.

A Cesarean is sometimes elected in advance in anticipation of a difficult and dangerous delivery, which may, in any case, end in an emergency Cesarean. While the decision between a vaginal delivery and an elective Cesarean is being made, doctors take account of a number of other factors. These include, in particular, the size and shape of the mother's pelvis, sometimes using an X-ray to help, the mother's blood pressure, age (it has been said that each decade of the mother's age adds another hour of labor), her general fitness and weight, the size of the baby, and the fetal heart function as demonstrated by the cardiotocograph. It is true to say that in this situation, as in almost any other affecting pregnancy, labor and delivery, all the details of the individual's case are considered. Individual variation can be very great, which is why the course of action for one woman may be quite different from the procedure adopted for another woman in an apparently similar situation.

BLEEDING

It was noted in Chapter 5 under *Hemorrhage* that two types of bleeding can occur in a pregnancy. One is concerned with the placenta and the other, incidental bleeding, occurs in a few pregnancies and often does not signify that there is anything to worry about. However, because some types of bleeding precede serious problems, you should always inform your doctor of any bleeding without delay.

In later pregnancy, with which this chapter is concerned, bleeding is described as antepartum hemorrhage, unless it is of the incidental type which may well have occurred at any time in the pregnancy. Antepartum hemorrhage has two main causes, both concerned with the placenta, in conditions known as placenta previa and placental abruption. (Although both conditions can occur in late pregnancy, it is also possible earlier, before the 28th week.)

Placenta previa

It happens in about 1 in 200 pregnancies that the placenta, from which the baby derives its nourishment and oxygen, instead of being attached shortly after conception near the baby at the upper part of the uterus, attaches further down by the cervix. As the placenta grows, it may eventually, in later pregnancy, cover the cervix, making normal delivery of the baby difficult but not impossible.

A sign of placenta previa is intermittent bleeding without pain; an ultrasound scan is used to determine the position of the placenta. In severe degrees of placenta previa, a Cesarean delivery is elected and, in the rare less serious cases, vaginal delivery can be achieved safely, if the birth canal allows passage of the baby's head without excessive bleeding.

Placental abruption (Abruptio placentae)

There will be some pain, if not severe pain, in this condition and this symptom is what distinguishes it from placenta previa. Part of the placenta, which in *abruptio* is in the normal place, detaches itself from the wall of the uterus, usually with pain and bleeding. In some cases, there is pain and no obvious bleeding from the vagina; in others there is severe pain and bleeding. One in three cases of placental abruption is associated with raised blood pressure and pre-eclampsia.

Once the placenta starts to detach itself, in placental abruption, labor must be induced right away or an emergency Cesarean performed in order to save the baby, which depends for its life upon the nourishment and oxygen brought to it by the placenta. If the abruption is small and the baby very premature, very careful observation in a hospital high-risk unit may be advised. One in three cases of placental abruption is associated with raised blood pressure and pre-eclampsia.

PREMATURE RUPTURE OF MEMBRANES (PROM)

Normally, the membranes surrounding the baby in the uterus rupture at the onset of labor. Usually known as the water bag breaking, this is entirely painless. The water may break some time before labor starts, and, in that case, you may be admitted to the hospital for rest and to prevent infection or damage to the baby. If the water has not broken and you are already in labor, it is sometimes broken by a doctor if the head is well engaged. This artificial rupture of the membranes is known as AROM. It is said that breaking the water can result in a shorter labor, which is normally a good thing for both mother and baby, provided that delivery is not so fast as to be explosive. When the membranes rupture of their own accord, this is noted on your records as spontaneous rupture of membranes (SROM).

The "water" refers to the liquid contained within the membranes that surround the baby. The liquid is composed of amniotic fluid (clear yellowish liquid) which contains the baby's urine and skin cells. Breaking the water means breaking the membranes that surround and protect the baby in the uterus. These membranes, the chorion and the amnion, protect the baby from the outside environment and particularly from infection, other than substances or infections that can cross the placenta from the mother's body to the baby's. The membranes can break spontaneously, in preparation for the birth of the baby, or they can be broken (ruptured) by the doctor by a device called an amnihook, which looks like a crochet hook, either in preparation for birth where labor is advanced or prior to an induction.

The baby is dependent for its well-being in the uterus on amniotic fluid for the following reasons: the baby can move about; the fluid distends the uterus so that the walls do not exert pressure upon the baby; the fluid and the membranes guarantee a constant temperature for the baby (i.e., the mother's body temperature); the fluid absorbs the baby's waste products; and it acts as a shock absorber for the baby. While the baby is floating freely in the liquid, it is protected not only from pressure from the uterine walls but also from outside pressure and from the impact, for example, of any fall or blow sustained by the mother. For all these reasons, once the water has broken hospital admission or bedrest is highly desirable.

The water normally breaks with an unmistakable gush of liquid, from which you may wish to protect yourself when out by wearing a sanitary pad and when in bed with a rubber sheet beneath the bottom sheet. Occasionally, however, the water breaks less unmistakably so that it can be difficult to distinguish it from the characteristic incontinence, or involuntary urination, of pregnancy. If you are in any doubt, telephone your doctor and, in the meantime, rest. The hospital can perform simple, quick tests to differentiate between amniotic fluid and urine. They can also tell if you are in labor by checking the dilation of your cervix (see figure 8, p. 131).

INDUCTION

Labor can be induced artificially at the hospital if it has become apparent that the baby needs to be born without delay but there is no sign of labor contractions starting. This is known as induction. One way of inducing labor is by rupturing the membranes, as we have seen above. Once this is done, contractions usually start fairly soon.

There are two other methods of inducing labor and delivery, by prostaglandin gel and by syntocinon drip. Only the drip is widely available in the United States.

Reasons for induction

There are many reasons for considering an induction and these include:

1. Pre-eclampsia in the woman. If the condition is advanced or resistant to treatment, it is essential to deliver the baby as quickly as possible.

2. High blood pressure in the woman, partly because high blood pressure is associated with pre-eclampsia and partly because it can be a dangerous condition in itself.
3. The condition of the placenta. When the pregnancy has completed its 42nd week—in other words—it is post-mature, there is a risk that the placenta will have out-grown its value to the baby. This may be confirmed either by scan or cardiotocography (see Chapter 9) and induction may be indicated. Because of the risks of post-maturity to the baby, many obstetricians would induce labor at the completion of the 42nd week, if not a little before.
4. The diabetic mother. Babies of diabetics are at risk of still birth in the last weeks of pregnancy, so delivery is normally advised before 40 weeks. Some diabetic women also develop hyptertension, another indication for induction (see 2 above).
5. In rhesus-negative women with antibodies, in whom delivery must be managed carefully, with the relevant specialists all available. In some cases of rhesus incompatibility, the baby may need a complete change of blood; clearly, this is better done when specialists, supplies and equipment are all easily accessible.
6. A small-for-dates baby, whatever the cause. If it is clearly failing to thrive, many consultants agree it is better to deliver the baby and treat it, in intensive care if necessary.
7. An overdue baby. Babies are routinely induced if they are more than two weeks overdue for two chief reasons: firstly, the placenta is likely to be exhausted and not providing the baby with much oxygen; secondly, the baby is growing and growing, and the bones of its head becoming firmer day by day. This means, as each day passes, the delivery will become more difficult for the mother and increasingly stressful for the baby as it pushes its way out. Not only is the head growing larger, but it is also becoming firmer and more resistant to the pressure it would normally experience as it descends the birth canal. There is also the mother's blood pressure and her general condition to take into account in prolonged pregnancies. A previous stillbirth would be another strong reason for not wishing a baby to become overdue.

Syntocinon drip

In the United States, the syntocinon drip is the most widely used method. Syntocinon is the synthetic version of oxytocin, a hormone released by the body at the onset of labor. Diluted syntocinon is given in an intravenous solution via a drip into a vein until regular contractions are established, with the amount administered increased as necessary. The baby's condition and the contractions need to be monitored; in other words, continuous internal fetal monitoring is required.

The syntocinon drip encourages the natural forces of labor, once labor has begun. However, if the cervix is "unripe" (thick and closed), this method is relatively inefficient at starting labor.

Some women feel that the syntocinon drip can make contractions very strong and painful, but others have no adverse reaction. The syntocinon drip is used with or without AROM.

Prostaglandin gel

A relatively new induction procedure in the United States is prostaglandin gel, which can be applied directly to the cervix.

This method is more useful than syntocinon in ripening a closed cervix and beginning the labor process. The synthetic hormone imitates the natural prostaglandins which the body releases during labor, bringing a gentler, more natural action. However, it is not universally available. It is widely used in Great Britain.

Some people favor prostaglandin induction because it leaves the woman free to move about in labor. This is not possible with syntocinon as a drip has to be used. Others prefer syntocinon because, should intravenous fluids—such as glucose and salt—be required, the drip is already in place.

Other methods of induction

Castor oil with a warm enema is something of the past, being both unnecessary and unpleasant. There are also a number of other methods of induction, none of which can be recommended. Induction should be carried out only under medical supervision in a properly equipped hospital.

Problems with induction

Many women believe that induction will lead to a shorter, more painful labor with more powerful contractions and that pain relief, which may deaden the senses, will be required as a consequence of the induction. In fact, this is not necessarily so, provided that the amount of synthetic hormone administered is correct.

It is true that induction is often associated with continuous fetal monitoring, either externally or internally, and that this monitoring restricts movement, and in turn may cause labor to become both painful and prolonged. Because of this, pain relief in the form of an epidural may be required. Inductions are also often associated with a forceps delivery and a cut (episiotomy). However, it is not induction itself that is responsible for these associated medical interventions: It is the reasons for the induction that are responsible. Labor and delivery of diabetic women, who often have to be induced, have to be closely supervised and this means continuous fetal monitoring. In cases of mild cephalo-pelvic disproportion, as another example, delivery by forceps and episiotomy may hasten delivery after a long labor, which at times may be best for mother or baby.

Inductions are timed for the convenience of medical and nursing staff so that delivery occurs not at three in the morning, when no one is at their best, but before the end of the hospital's normal day. The nursing staff work in shifts, but the doctor stays with you. If inductions were not timed for a reasonable hour, it could often mean that a doctor was on duty all day and then up for another 8 to 10 hours or so, in other words, right through the night. It is when people are tired that mistakes are made. Clearly, emergencies require a senior obstetrician to be called, but there is no medical need to allow deliveries that require induction or close medical supervision to take place in the middle of the night.

To what extent inductions have been carried out for a combination of medical and practical reasons as outlined above compared with those performed for purely "social" reasons can only be judged by assessing each individual case. Social reasons are very often dictated by the woman's domestic requirements, rather than the requirements of medical and nursing staff.

If you do not understand fully the reasons that an induction is being proposed, ask for the reasons to be explained to you.

The majority of births in the United States are performed by obstetricians in hospitals. Uncomplicated births may be attended by nurse-midwives or family practitioners. A small percentage of births occur at home for a variety of reasons. Some are carefully planned home births which parents prefer for philosophical reasons. Others are not so carefully planned home births that occur there due to financial reasons.

Most health care professionals would like to see hospital routines become flexible enough to enable all women to feel comfortable in a hospital setting, as well as universal maternity benefits available to the poor, who may not be able to afford hospital delivery.

CESAREAN SECTION

Approximately one in four babies is born by Cesarean section rather than vaginally. In some private hospitals the rate can be as high as 40 percent.

A Cesarean section is performed by making an incision along the bikini line and lifting the baby out. This operation, which is in fact major surgery, is performed either under general anesthetic or with a spinal or an epidural. It takes between 5 and 10 minutes to make the incision and deliver the baby and a further 35 to 40 minutes to stitch the cut.

An elective Cesarean is one for which the need has been decided in advance; an emergency Cesarean is the same operation carried out when the woman is already in labor and it becomes clear that there is an urgent need to deliver the baby quickly (see *Reasons for a Cesarean* further on).

Anesthetics for Cesarean section

The operation is performed either with a regional (spinal or epidural) or under general anesthetic. It is now generally agreed that a regional, in which the mother is conscious but unable to feel pain, is by far the better choice. If it is working properly, the mother can feel sensation but not pain and is fully awake. It means, moreover, that the baby can be handed to her soon after it is delivered and it can begin to breast feed (provided that there are no complications of the sort that indicate the child needs special care directly). It also means that the woman's partner may remain with her, which in most hospitals he cannot do if the operation is performed under general anesthetic.

In a spinal anesthetic, a small amount of local anesthetic is placed in the spinal fluid. In an epidural anesthetic, the local anesthetic is placed in the space around the spinal fluid, the "epidural space." Spinal anesthetics are quicker and more reliable but there is a small chance of a spinal headache.

Recovery from an epidural is quicker than from a general anesthetic and it can also be topped up if the woman indicates to the anesthesiologist that she is feeling pain. There will be less postoperative pain with regional as compared with a general anesthetic and the baby will suffer less effect from regional than from a full anesthetic. Lastly, the mother will be up and around more quickly after a Cesarean performed with regional than a Cesarean under general anesthetic. For all these reasons, most doctors prefer to offer a spinal or an epidural, although some women are, understandably, initially wary of agreeing to undergo major surgery while awake.

Choosing between a spinal or an epidural and a general anesthetic   It is clear that it is preferable to have a Cesarean with an epidural rather than a general anesthetic. However, if the operation has to be performed as an emergency, you can only have it by epidural if the instruments are already set up. If you have elected to try labor without an epidural, and it subsequently proves impossible or dangerous to continue towards a vaginal delivery, you may have to have the Cesarean under general anesthetic if there is not time to set up an epidural. Because of this, if you have been advised that you can try for vaginal delivery but that it may turn out that the baby has to be delivered by Cesarean, it may be wise to accept an epidural, as the risks with this are lower than with

general anesthetic. In any case, don't eat anything once you know you are in labor.

An increasing number of Cesareans, and in some hospitals the vast majority, are performed with an epidural, whether they are elective or emergency operations. The figure might be higher if it were not for the fact that an epidural requires an experienced anesthesiologist to be in constant attendance, and this cannot always be arranged, particularly if it is an emergency Cesarean. In some small hospitals an anesthesiologist is available only on certain days or at certain times. The choice between a spinal or an epidural may depend upon the skill and experience of the anesthesiologist or anesthetist.

Reasons for a Cesarean

Firstly, a Cesarean is performed only when it is considered either dangerous or impossible, either for the mother or the baby, for the baby to be safely delivered vaginally. The reasons include:

1. a prolonged labor (which may happen for a number of reasons, including the fact that it is a first baby; the baby's head is too big for the mother's pelvis; or the baby is in an unusual position)
2. slow or inert labor ("inert" meaning that labor started but did not progress)
3. labor not starting and induction fails
4. breech presentation (as described earlier in this chapter)
5. placenta previa (in which the placenta is lying across the cervix and would be ruptured if labor was allowed to continue, causing dangerous bleeding, known as antepartum hemorrhage)
6. the baby is short of oxygen and thus becoming distressed to a degree where its well-being is threatened
7. a mother with severe pre-eclampsia, or eclampsia
8. pelvic tumors, such as fibroids or ovarian cysts, obstructing the baby's delivery
9. previous stillbirth or previous complicated and difficult delivery
10. the baby has assumed an oblique or transverse lie
11. any risk delivery, including forceps deliveries, when Cesarean presents more acceptable (i.e. lower) risks

A second or subsequent Cesarean

The situation should be no more complicated, provided that proper care is given, if you have had your first child by Cesarean and you are now pregnant for the second or subsequent time. It is now no longer the case that "once a Cesarean, always a Cesarean." Whether or not you will need a Cesarean for second and subsequent pregnancies depends on the reasons for the first Cesarean. For example, if the reason was cephalo-pelvic disproportion, then a second Cesarean may very well be required. Again, if the cervix failed to dilate, it may fail to do so again. If, on the other hand, the cause was placenta previa or breech, and this time the placenta is in a suitable position to allow the baby to be born vaginally, or the second baby is not breech, there is no reason to elect a Cesarean.

In the old days, many women believed that if the first child was born by Cesarean, then the next would be as well, and, in addition, that only two such operations could be performed and therefore that their family must be limited to two. However, it is perfectly possible to have several Cesarean deliveries, although most experts believe that three to four is enough and you may well be discouraged from having more than this. To perform second and subsequent Cesareans, the original scar is reopened and used again, so that you are left with only one scar. Because the scar implies an area of potential weakness in the uterus, most obstetricians would advise a wait of a year before the next conception.

It is possible to have a vaginal delivery of a second or subsequent child after a first Cesarean and there is no reason why the labor may not be perfectly normal. However, any bleeding or lower abdominal pain may indicate some weakness in the scar and should be reported to your doctor without delay. The type of uterine incision a woman has had in the past is important. Most Cesarean sections are done through the lower uterine segment, with a horizontal incision. Such an incision is unlikely to cause problems. However, occasionally, Cesarean sections are done vertically and high along the uterine wall. This "classical incision" has a higher chance of rupturing, should the woman go into labor. Women who have a vertical incision should schedule their Cesarean sections well before labor can occur. Labor cannot be allowed to become prolonged with a second or subsequent child because it places a strain upon the Cesarean scar. An episiotomy may be performed in order to facilitate a prompt delivery. (Incidentally, the scar from the Cesarean delivery of the first child ruptures only in extremely rare cases when labor has been allowed to become prolonged and in which the contractions are extremely powerful.) If labor does appear to be prolonged, an emergency Cesarean may have to be performed, but, as was noted above, this does not prevent you having successive Cesarean sections up to a maximum of 4. Overall, 60%–80% of women with prior Cesareans can deliver vaginally if allowed to try. Unfortunately, many obstetricians do not encourage women to have a VBAC (vaginal birth after Cesarean) due to concerns about liability if problems should occur. Many women, as well, do not want a trial of labor depending upon the circumstances of their first Cesarean section. They may dread the recurrence of a long, painful labor and a frightening birth experience.

WHAT TO TAKE WITH YOU

This chapter has been concerned with the last four weeks of pregnancy and has therefore described what you may be feeling, the routine checks of weeks 36 to 40, false labor and the baby's position. However, this chapter has also had to cover induction and elective Cesareans as these are often performed before your estimated date of delivery. The sort of complications likely to make either of these procedures necessary may have been apparent for some weeks, but it is only now, ideally after the 37th week, that either induction or Cesarean can be performed. Both procedures can be carried out earlier if it is felt medically desirable either for the mother or the baby.

With these things in mind it is well worth packing a small case containing all the things you will need for a few days well ahead of your estimated date of delivery—it is, after all, only an estimated date, and it is very common to go into labor a week or two before the predicted date. Your case should include bathrobe, slippers, nightgowns (that open down the front if you intend to breast feed), comfortable loose clothes and underclothes (including a nursing bra), something to read, toiletries (including toothbrush and toothpaste, shampoo, deodorant), cosmetics, address and telephone book. Check with your hospital to see if you will need a telephone credit card or may need change for a pay phone. Think, too, about anything you might like to have with you while you are in labor.

GIVING BIRTH AT HOME

It may now be clearer, if you have read all the previous chapters of the book, why little has been said about home births. The main objection made by doctors to home births is that if any unforeseen complication arises, in what seemed to be a straightforward pregnancy, the time lost in conveying the mother to the hospital may threaten not only her life but the life of the baby. A straightforward birth is a retrospective diagnosis: No one knows until after the event if it is straightforward or otherwise.

Any woman who is in a high-risk category (refer to the Table of Positive Risk Factors in Chapter 6) will be delivered in the hospital with access to the different types of specialist (heart, kidney, anesthesiologist, pediatrician, etc.) and to all the facilities that a modern, well-equipped hospital can offer, a neonatal intensive care unit being just one of those facilities.

It is perfectly possible, and indeed it is the norm, to have a low-tech delivery in a high-tech hospital environment. If you wish to minimize interventions and hospital routines, pick your doctor or midwife and hospital very carefully to be certain they will support your decision. Explore early discharge options and family-centered birthing units.

Many doctors sympathize and understand very well the reasons why some women would prefer to be delivered at home. They feel, however, that their responsibility is to both the mother and the child, and they can fulfill this responsibility better if they are given the opportunity to work in the place where they usually work, with the full array of equipment, and access to specialists in other disciplines if a crisis arises.

Lastly, if you already have one child or more, it may prove difficult or even distressing for them to hear you in labor, although there is no doubt they will be thrilled when they see the newborn baby. You will probably feel tired, and yet feel compelled to carry on with the running of the house and looking after your existing children. If you intend to give birth at home, therefore, do make sure there is someone to look after you and to take over household routines. You may not want to have to answer the telephone or the doorbell within a day of giving birth to your baby.

If you do opt for a home birth, find out what would happen to you in an emergency. Some (the better) home birth attendants have formal backup arrangements with hospitals; others simply tell you to go to the emergency room and leave you on your own.

Giving birth in the hospital is the subject of the next chapter.

11. Giving Birth

The time has almost arrived for you to give birth to your baby. Many women feel at this time a sense of elation and anticipation combined with apprehension about the processes of the birth. You will be feeling confident, however, about what lies ahead because you have followed the details of your pregnancy with an informed interest and have been able to ask the right questions at the right time. Knowing what is happening to you, to the baby, and the reasons for various medical procedures all helps to make you feel happy and secure. Don't forget in these final stages to ask the medical or nursing staff about anything that puzzles you.

HOW WILL I KNOW?

Very many women worry about whether or not they will recognize the signs of impending labor and conjure up visions of having to deliver on a bus or in a taxi! This is a common worry, but only in exceptionally rare cases does it happen and usually only then to women who did not known what to expect.

There are a number of important signs which indicate that your labor is probably starting and that you should be taken to hospital. These include your water bag breaking, a "show," and contractions becoming both regular and pronounced, and probably painful. If your water breaks (signifying that the membranes surrounding the baby in the uterus have ruptured) or if you have had a pinkish show of blood, you should be taken to the hospital. If you have contractions, but you have had no show and the water has not broken, you may wish to telephone the hospital in order to confirm that you should go in. In the last week or so of pregnancy, it is possible to confuse the Braxton Hicks contractions of late pregnancy (described in the previous chapter) with the genuine contractions of the first stage of labor. In other words, then, the three important signs of labor can occur independently of each other or in combination: It is quite possible to be in the first stage of labor, with fairly pronounced contractions, even though the water has not broken.

Not going too soon

Some women delay going to the hospital for as long as possible in the belief that this will save them long, boring hours in the labor ward and that medical assistance and monitoring will consequently be reduced to a minimum. There is probably something to be said for the first reason, but the second is illogical. If someone needs medical assistance, they will receive it either in a relaxed atmosphere, if there is plenty of time, or as an emergency room procedure.

Clearly, no one wants to be admitted and then discharged because they are in fact in false labor, but doctors agree that they would prefer to have a few cases of false labor than a rushed, last-minute admission in which the baby arrives within minutes of the mother walking through the doors of the hospital.

If you are in any doubt, do not hesitate to call the hospital and discuss your condition with someone on the labor ward: They will be sympathetic and understanding. They will probably ask you how long you have felt the contractions, at what intervals they are coming, and have you had a "show." Once they have the information, they will be able to advise you.

Don't leave it till the last minute

Putting off going to the hospital until the last minute is not a wise thing to do. If, for example, the traffic is held up—by an accident, by the rush hour, or by an obstruction on the road—you may find yourself well into the second stage of labor, with the baby's arrival imminent, and the hospital still a long way off. If even a minor complication occurs at this point, your health and that of your baby's could be threatened. The chance is simply not worth taking. It is far better to spend an extra hour or two at the hospital than to create this sort of situation, which can prove alarming if not actually dangerous.

ADMISSION TO THE HOSPITAL

When you arrive at the hospital, you will go through the normal admissions procedure, involving administrative matters, and your record will be located. You will then be taken to the labor ward where you will undress and be given various checks. Your pulse, temperature and blood pressure will be taken and you will be examined both externally and internally in order to judge the baby's position and to see how far the cervix (the neck of the uterus) has dilated in preparation for the baby's birth. (See Figure 8.)

The stomach becomes much less efficient while you are in labor and it is therefore difficult to empty the bowels. Because of this, you may be offered suppositories or an enema, in order to relieve internal pressure, but you do not have to accept either if you don't want to. However, you should not eat now as this will obviously increase any sense of fullness; in addition, if an emergency Cesarean became necessary, the anesthesiologist would be faced with the possibility of you vomiting under anesthetic and inhaling the vomit—a very dangerous situation. The urge to vomit can be suppressed by drugs, however.

Hospitals used to shave pregnant women as a matter of routine, but this is no longer done unless a Cesarean is to be performed. If shaving is proposed for a normal vaginal delivery, you may refuse it if you wish, since there is little point to it.

YOUR BIRTH PLAN

It is the routine practice of many hospitals these days to discuss with you a birth plan at one of your visits to the office or clinic. This is a plan on which are noted your wishes and feelings about your labor and delivery: It may include a note of who you would like to be present; what position you hope to adopt for labor and delivery; your feelings about fetal monitoring, both external and internal; induction; episiotomy; pain relief—do you wish to have any, and if so what sort; whether or not you wish to have the baby on your chest immediately after delivery before it is cleaned up; whether you intend to feed by breast or bottle, and whether or not you intend to feed on demand; your feelings about a stay in the hospital; and so on.

You can guess by the nature of the topics on the birth plan that such a plan can at best only be a plan rather than an agenda of what is actually going to happen. Labor and delivery take their own direction in each individual case, acquiring a momentum of their own; It depends just what happens in any particular case whether or not the birth plan can be adhered to. Equally, you may change your mind about certain things. For example, you may wish to avoid an episiotomy: However, if the baby becomes severely distressed and needs to be delivered quickly with forceps, an episiotomy may have to be performed. To give another example, some women would prefer to have a "natural" childbirth with no pain relief. It is not possible, however, to predict the degree of pain that may occur nor any individual's pain threshold—in other words, how much pain she can stand.

The birth plan, then, is a provisional plan. You may deviate from it if you wish, and the medical and nursing staff will do so if

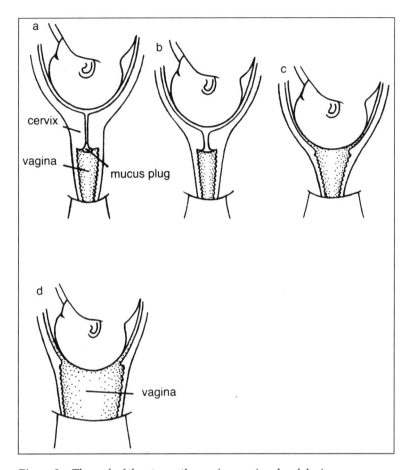

Figure 8. *The neck of the uterus, the cervix, remains closed during pregnancy and is sealed by a mucus plug (see a). Shortly before the onset of labor, the cervix starts to shorten (see b) in response to the contractions. A partially dilated cervix (see c), now encouraged by the pressure of the baby's head, is one of the signs that labor is well under way and can easily be recognized by medical and nursing staff. By the time the cervix has dilated or opened out sufficiently to allow the passage of the baby's head through into the vagina (see d), the second stage of labor has been reached and the baby's delivery could now be very rapid.*

circumstances dictate that it is medically desirable to do so in the interests of your health and that of the baby.

MONITORING

The baby's heart rate can be recorded electronically by means of fetal monitoring. The action of the baby's heart rate is the best measurement there is of the baby's well-being in labor. If the baby's heart rate decreases, it signifies that the baby is not receiving enough oxygen, on which its well-being and ultimately its life depend. The decrease in heart beat will appear on the cardiotocogram as explained in Chapter 9. The baby may not be receiving sufficient oxygen for two reasons: (1) because the umbilical cord that connects the baby with the placenta has become depressed; or (2) because the oxygen coming from the placenta is insufficient.

If the baby's heart rate remains slow in labor for any reason for several minutes (a long time in this context), some of its brain cells may die off and this may result in some serious impairment either in the form of physical handicap or mental handicap. The baby's heart normally beats at between 120 and 160 beats per minute; "slow" in this context, therefore, means less than 90 beats per minute. The cause for decreased heart rate is clearly important and it was for this reason that the fetal blood sampling technique was developed. Analysis of a blood sample indicates whether an insufficient supply of oxygen is caused by an intermittent, recoverable problem, such as cord compression, or whether it is caused by a chronic problem with the placenta providing insufficient oxygen (caused by placental insufficiency or other problems associated with the mother's blood flow).

How the baby's heartbeat is monitored
Electronic fetal heart monitoring can be carried out externally by means of a transducer and belt affixed to the mother's abdomen, or internally by affixing an electrode by means of a tiny clip in the skin of the baby's scalp or buttocks. The external monitor can be taken on and off easily, allowing medical and nursing staff to check from time to time that the baby's heart is beating regularly; or it can be left on for continuous monitoring, which is particularly desirable in high-risk pregnancies. The internal monitor, once applied, has to be left in place for the duration of labor and therefore provides continuous monitoring.

There is also a new form of continuous fetal monitoring, known as telemetry. Unlike those systems in current use, telemetry allows you to walk about. You have a battery strapped to your thigh, which transmits messages from the probe attached to your abdomen or the baby's scalp. It works on the same principle as a remote control device for a television. This is already available in some hospitals and will become more widely available. As well as this more acceptable form of internal continuous fetal monitoring, telemetry may in the future be used for continuous external monitoring at home, prior to labor.

Advantages of electronic monitoring
No other method gives such a precise and sensitive assessment of the baby's heart rate, and thus its condition as labor progresses

towards delivery. The baby receives its vital oxygen from the placenta. Each time a contraction comes, the blood vessels of the uterus are constricted and this causes a temporary reduction in the supply of oxygenated blood to the baby. This temporary reduction does not adversely affect the baby as it will have enough oxygen in reserve. However, if the oxygen supply is more reduced, or if the baby for whatever reason has less in reserve, the baby may be starved of oxygen, with potentially disastrous consequences.

Disadvantages of electronic monitoring

External monitoring depends for accurate results on the equipment being properly located, and if the baby moves about this is affected. Internal monitoring requires the probe to be fixed to the baby's scalp, but this has not been known to cause any long-lasting damage to the baby. Claims concerning injuries, infections and abscesses have been greatly exaggerated: There is not usually any problem with fetal electrodes. It is possible that those worried about fetal electrodes may have confused this technique with fetal blood sampling, which can be more hazardous. However, women with HIV (AIDS) infections should avoid scalp electrodes, if possible, to avoid puncture of the baby's scalp.

Machines characteristically go wrong at times, and, in addition, electrical interference can make it difficult to interpret the printout correctly. Doctors and midwives are well aware of these hazards and the machinery is therefore checked, before further action is taken, if the printout indicates gross changes in the baby's heart rate.

If your baby is being monitored continuously, you will not be able to walk about, unless telemetry is available, which can be irritating if you are in labor for several hours. Moreover, in certain positions, the blood flow may decrease and labor may then become prolonged. This can create a vicious circle in which the baby becomes distressed because the labor has been prolonged as a result of using equipment designed to identify such distress. For this reason, many doctors believe in the happy medium of on and off monitoring for apparently normal pregnancies and labors.

If you are immobilized upon a bed, you are not free to move about. When the mother is lying down, the main vein and artery in her back are compressed, which hinders optimum blood flow, and this causes the blood pressure to drop. For these reasons, if you are to be continuously monitored, and therefore immobilized, you will be asked to turn to one side and supported with a wedge so that you cannot lie flat on your back. However, the monitor can be used in a variety of positions, including standing, squatting or on hands and knees, presuming your attendant is willing to adjust the monitor frequently as you change positions.

For high-risk pregnancies, most doctors support continuous fetal monitoring in the latter part of the first stage of labor and accept that such monitoring has certain hazards—again, this is a question of risk-benefit ratio. High-risk pregnancies in this context include very premature labors, induced labors (depending upon the reason for the induction), and in pregnancies in which complications, such as raised blood pressure, diabetes, vaginal bleeding or a small-for-dates baby, are known to exist. The risk-benefit ratio, in which the risks of continuous monitoring must be weighed against the benefits that it can offer both mother and baby, must be considered.

FETAL DISTRESS

Monitoring the baby's heartbeat is intended to identify fetal distress (which can be confirmed by fetal blood sampling), so that the appropriate steps may be taken to help the baby. "Distress" in this context means something much more serious than "upset." Fetal distress is the term used to indicate that the baby is receiving insufficient oxygen, on which it depends for its well-being and ultimately its life. The baby receives oxygen from the mother's blood through the medium of the placenta. If there is something wrong with the placenta, as in the case of *placental insufficiency*, *placenta previa* or *placental abruption*, the amount of oxygen transferred is reduced. The baby may consequently become increasingly starved of oxygen and it is at this point that appropriate action must be taken.

If you or I become short of oxygen (panting, breathless and with aches in the muscles), we can stop whatever it is we are doing and take in large gulps of air (oxygen). The unborn baby cannot, of course, do this and, in addition, it may be in an environment in which the oxygen supply is already lower than it ought to be for the baby's health. If the baby becomes short of oxygen, it will not be long before the brain cells start to die off. The brain cells do not repair themselves and thus this permanent damage leads to spasticity and mental impairment in the baby.

One way of identifying fetal distress, once labor has started and the water has broken, is by the appearance of the baby's waste products at the vagina. What happens is this: Oxygen starvation stimulates what is known as the vagus, the vagal nerve. When this happens to the baby, the heartbeat becomes faster, there is an increase in blood circulation and there is also bowel activity. The baby opens its bowel and excretes waste matter. Because the water has broken (in other words, the membranes surrounding the baby have ruptured), this waste matter eventually appears at the vagina. This matter is known as meconium and is a very dark green color.

If the presence of meconium is detected at the vagina, it proves that the baby either has suffered a recent shortage of oxygen or is still suffering from a shortage. In order to work out which it is, in other words whether the baby is still distressed, doctors look at the cardiotocograph or take a fetal blood sample.

Another sign of fetal distress, which can occur during pregnancy or labor, is the baby turning over and over with sudden or violent movements. If this should happen, the obstetrician will decide how best to deliver the baby immediately. Occasionally, signs of fetal distress are detected before the start of labor. For instance, fetal monitoring during an at-risk pregnancy at one of the visits to the prenatal clinic may reveal worrying signs on the heart tracing (beat-to-beat variations as described in Chapter 9). This would mean that the baby may have to be delivered before term (before its EDC), either by inducing labor or by a Cesarean.

BABY'S BLOOD TEST

A sample of the baby's blood, known as fetal blood sampling, can be taken from its scalp while it is still in the uterus. This is done only in labor, after the membranes have ruptured, and only if problems which merit further investigation present themselves (such as decreased heart rate signifying an insufficiency in the oxygen supply to the baby).

If a lack of oxygen exists, acid is produced. It is this acid that kills off the brain cells. This is why it is essential to know why the lack of oxygen has occurred—whether the cause is intermittent and recoverable, or chronic. If we exercise in an unaccustomedly vigorous fashion, our muscles ache. This ache is caused by the release of lactic acid, the acid that is produced in response to a lack of oxygen. As it was said earlier, if this happens to us, we can stop doing whatever we are doing and take in gulps of air. The unborn baby cannot do this, and must therefore be assisted without delay.

How the baby's blood is sampled

An amnioscope (which works in a similar fashion to the telescope) is inserted into the vagina. A minute needle is passed through the amnioscope to withdraw no more than a drop of the baby's blood from its scalp. The needle is tiny, smaller than those used for taking a drop of blood from the thumb prior to donating blood, and not unlike those used in home blood sugar test kits for diabetics. The baby's blood is tested and the results often prove invaluable in the successful management of high-risk pregnancies. If a lack of oxygen is confirmed, a Cesarean delivery may be done. It should be noted that fetal blood sampling is carried out only when there is already reason to suspect that something is amiss.

The technique can, very occasionally, lead to the baby developing a minor, localized infection on the scalp but should not cause any serious or long-lasting damage.

MIND OVER MATTER

This chapter has so far discussed knowing when to go to the hospital, and the subject of fetal monitoring, and the reasons for such monitoring. As labor progresses, pain relief sometimes becomes a priority. It was noted earlier in this chapter under the heading of *Your birth plan* that some women elect for a "natural" childbirth with no pain relief. There is no logical connection in this context between "natural" and "absence of pain." Cats, dogs and horses all give birth naturally, but they nevertheless experience pain in doing so.

The movement for "natural" childbirth, in which is implicit a rejection of all technology and drugs, has increased the expectations of some women of a delivery without pain. Some lucky women do have very little pain, but most experience some. Some of those who most fervently hoped "to do it all themselves," but who in the end accept relief from pain feel let down and to some degree inadequate. This is unnecessary, when one appreciates that natural childbirth always has and always will involve some degree of pain and discomfort.

It is true, however, that the movement for natural childbirth has proved valuable in several respects: Firstly, it has encouraged women to be aware of what is happening to them and has encouraged them to ask questions; secondly, it has removed some of the fear—a fear of the unknown—that women experience as they approach the time of delivery; thirdly, it has shown, more effectively than the medical profession has, that there exist non-medicinal ways of coping with the pain.

Fear of the unknown leads to tension, both of a physical and mental nature. Physical tension makes it impossible to relax and causes pain in the muscles. In this way pain is heightened, producing yet more fear and apprehension. It follows, therefore, that the more a woman feels in control of her body and of what is going on around her, the more relaxed and less fearful she will be. Feeling relaxed takes the edge off pain, which gives you the feeling you are coping well. This increases your confidence, which of course helps you to feel more relaxed.

There are women who may find that they cannot cope for the entire length of a long labor without some help. A first baby may take over 12 hours to appear and perhaps much longer. If the labor starts at any time after the early morning, therefore, this means being in labor, and thus awake, not only all through the day but most of the night as well. Women most likely to want relief from

Table 11.1 PAIN RELIEF: THE OPTIONS			
Stage of labor and delivery	**Prefer to do without pain relief, but may change mind**	**Want some pain relief**	**Want total pain relief**
1st stage of labor	—	Narcotic injection	Epidural
2nd stage of labor	— If, as labor progresses, you would like some relief, you can have a pudendal nerve block or caudal anaesthetic if a forceps delivery is indicated. Probably too late for an epidural. Too late for narcotic.	Pudendal nerve block for forceps delivery. Caudal.	Top up
Prolonged first stage of labor	Narcotic. Pethidine. Epidural. Paracervical block.	As above	Top up
Difficulties leading to emergency Cesarean delivery	General anesthetic, or epidural if still possible and if preferred.	General anesthetic, or epidural if still possible and if preferred.	Top up (in greatly increased quantity) thus avoiding general anesthetic if preferred.

pain are those who are having a long labor, those with a narrow pelvis, women with breech babies and women having their first baby. Methods of medical intervention used to be less reliable, and in the old days, therefore, labor was simply allowed to continue, sometimes for as long as 36 hours. This is a long time to be kept awake, and an even longer time to be awake *and* in pain.

There is no need, therefore, why any woman should feel she has somehow failed if she accepts medical assistance, whether it be in the form of pain relief, induction, or a Cesarean delivery. All these things are done with the interests of the mother and the baby foremost. Women who feel a sense of failure about the delivery of their baby are simply casualties of the more vociferous exponents of "natural" childbirth. Some people are simply "anti-doctor," resenting a doctor's air of authority. They may be particularly so in the context of giving birth, if that doctor is male, and some of them have found a useful outlet in the natural childbirth movement.

Table 11.2   CHOOSING PAIN RELIEF

Pain relief	How given	How long to work	Advantages	Disadvantages
Nitrous oxide and oxygen	You breath in from mouthpiece (similar to oxygen mask demonstrated by airline stewardesses)	15-20 seconds	Safe and simple	Not available in many hospitals. May make you feel light-headed or very sleepy. Difficult to put your breathing techniques into practice while using mask. Does not give complete relief from pain.
Narcotics, such as Demerol, Dilaudid, or morphine	Injection into a vein in your arm or into a muscle in your bottom	Up to 10 minutes. Peak effect at 30-60 minutes. Lasts for 1–3 hours.	Simple, can be quickly administered. Narcotic Antagonist may be given to baby if baby drowsy.	Timing of the injection is crucial: If it is given too early, it wears off before you really need it. If it is given less than 2 hours before delivery, you may not be able to push when you need to, which may lead to a forceps delivery. You may feel drowsy or high or detached. You may also feel nauseated. If the narcotic is given late, the baby may seem sleepy and slow to breathe, in which case it is given an injection to counter the effects of the narcotic. Only a certain amount of narcotic can be given because of its depressive effect upon the baby. Depresses cerebral function and baby may not be able to breathe. Then has to be intubated and forcibly oxygenated (by hand or by pump).
Pudendal nerve block	Injection through wall of vagina to block pudendal nerve	About 5-10 minutes. Lasts for about 20 minutes.	This is a local anesthetic which affects the vulva, vagina and perineum. Useful for short, second-state labor procedures, such as forceps delivery.	May not work. May depress baby and get danger amount of local anesthetic into
Para-cervical nerve block	Injection into cervix	5-10 minutes. Lasts for 1-2 hours.	Quick and simple	May depress baby and get dangerous amount of local anesthetic into baby's system.

Pain relief	How given	How long to work	Advantages	Disadvantages
Epidural analgesia/ anesthetic	Saline drip set up, and local anesthetic injected into epidural space between spinal cord and the backbone of the lumbar region (see figure 10).	15-20 minutes. Topped up as required.	At its best, it gives complete relief of pain with no loss of awareness of what is going on—unlike narcotics. Ideal for use in difficult, painful labors, particularly if they may end in Cesarean delivery because the epidural can be topped up, eliminating the need for a general anesthetic. Baby likely to be less affected by epidural than by narcotics or general anesthetic.	The nature of this highly technical procedure means that it does not always work, and that only a trained and highly competent anesthetist can do it and then should be available to attend labor and delivery. It should be done in the first state of labor, ideally. Chances of forceps and episiotomy are higher. You will need an intravenous drip, and possibly a catheter for the bladder. Continuous fetal monitoring is likely. You may feel numbness in your legs for some time after delivery and you may (rarely) have a headache.
Epidural analgesia/anesthetic is discussed in more detail on the following pages.				
Caudal analgesia/ anesthesia	Single injection of local anesthetic given into tip of spine, right down at the base, in the sacral, as opposed to lumbar, area.	5-10 minutes.	Caudal anesthesia affects the nerve roots lower down in the spine, and fewer are affected, so that the effect is more limited than epidural. Shorter acting than epidural. Very suitable for the few minutes' pain relief required for forceps delivery. Headache and problems with blood pressure less likely than with epidural. Easier to administer than epidural. Good pain relief for a short time and less "paralyzing" effect than epidural.	Does not always work and occasionally works only on one side. Woman experiences numbness in lower part of body, making it difficult for her to push. Normally given as a single dose, unlike epidural which is typically topped up. Unlike epidural, cannot be used for prolonged labor or Cesarean delivery.

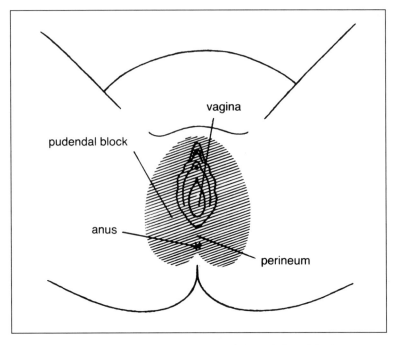

Figure 9. *A pudendal block, one of the forms of pain relief used during an assisted delivery, notably forceps or vacuum, anesthetizes the pudendal nerve. This local anesthetic affects the vulva, vagina and perineum as shown by the shaded area in the illustration.*

RELIEF FROM PAIN

So, there is absolutely no need to feel ashamed if you decide that you would like not to be in pain. There are several ways of approaching this, depending on your wishes, the degree of difficulty envisaged by doctors with your labor and delivery, and the types of relief available. You will see from the table above that, in hospital, there are different types of analgesia (pain relief) available: these include pudendal block (lidocaine); caudal anesthesia; epidural anesthesia; paracervical block anesthesia; and injections of narcotics, such as pethidine, morphine or Fortral. Occasionally, inhalation of a gas/oxygen mixture is used.

In order to combat pain you can also control your breathing, as you will have been taught either at childbirth preparation classes or by a childbirth instructor. Other complementary techniques include acupuncture and hypnosis, but for these you will have to arrange with the hospital in advance to have your own practitioner present throughout labor and delivery. Lastly, there is a fairly new method of pain relief known as TNS or TENS (transcutaneousnerve stimulation or transcutaneous electrical nerve stimulation). This comparatively new method is not yet widely available, and many mothers and doctors have reservations about its usefulness. It is thought to be without side effects, but many believe that it also without *any* effect. Many women derive no pain relief from it, and some doctors dismiss it, saying "Well, it doesn't do any harm, but it doesn't do much good, either." Some women have found it effective, however, and thus greatly preferable to the other types of pain relief available in hospitals that have side effects.

CHOOSING PAIN RELIEF

Choosing between the available options for pain relief in labor requires: a knowledge of what you think your pain threshold is; the degree of anticipated difficulty with your labor and delivery; and the advantages and disadvantages of each type of pain relief. Don't forget, too, the complementary techniques, which have proved successful for some women. Lastly, it should be understood that "total" pain relief can be something of a misnomer: Not all women are completely free of pain, even with an epidural.

EPIDURAL ANALGESIA AND ANESTHETIC

Table 11.2 on choosing pain relief gives a brief summary of the advantages and disadvantages of the different types of pain relief. As many women are unsure whether or not to have an epidural, and what its effects may be, it is worth taking a more detailed look at this specialized form of pain relief and anesthetic. Epidurals, incidentally, are routinely used in gynecological and orthopedic operations, and are therefore not confined to obstetrics.

When an epidural is given successfully, it can give spectacular pain relief in a normal labor, and it can provide effective anesthesia in complicated labor and delivery. It can also be a safer alternative to general anesthesia in Cesarean delivery. It is in effect a local anesthetic and therefore medically preferable to narcotics, which affect the baby as well as the mother, and general anesthesia which carries with it a variety of risks. Chief of these is the risk that the laboring woman may have eaten and the contents of the stomach may be regurgitated upwards through the esophagus, across into the trachea and down into the lungs, causing respiratory failure and death. This is associated more with emergency Cesareans, rather than planned Cesareans, for with the latter the mother is told not to eat or drink for 12 hours before the operation. Safety procedures will be followed in any case (see page 147).

How an epidural is given

First, a saline IV is set up so that fluid can be given into the bloodstream via a vein before the epidural, which should be administered only in the first stage of labor. A small plastic needle is inserted into a vein in the arm and the saline fluid infused. This is done in order to counteract a possible drop in the mother's blood pressure, sometimes caused by the injection of the local anesthetic, which may make the woman feel faint and sick, and the baby possibly distressed. Next, continuous fetal monitoring is set up, so that the baby's heart can be constantly assessed as it responds to the effect of the epidural upon its mother. If, for example, the mother's blood pressure dips, the baby receives less oxygen from the placenta. If this "starving" of oxygen was allowed to continue, it would have serious consequences. For these reasons, the baby's heart is monitored continuously and the mother's blood pressure checked every five minutes.

Once these steps have been taken, the epidural can be administered. (See Figure 10.) You will be asked to curl up into a ball, presenting your back to the anesthesiologist, or sit upon one side of the bed. The back is swabbed with spirit solution to make the area sterile. You must keep still when the epidural needle is to be inserted. The anesthesiologist then injects local anesthetic under the skin of the back so that the epidural needle causes the minimum amount of pain. The epidural needle is then injected into the epidural space between the spinal cord and the bones of the back, during which time it is essential that you keep still. Once the needle is in place, a tube (epidural catheter) is threaded down the needle and the needle is removed. The epidural catheter is fixed with sticky tape to your back. Provided that all is well, anesthetic is then passed down the tube from where it enters the epidural space and soon anesthetizes all the nerves in the area, giving good pain relief within about 20 minutes. A bladder catheter is sometimes also provided, as the anesthetic prevents control of the bladder.

Many women have wondered if it is safe to inject an area so close to the spinal cord. The chances of anything going wrong are very, very slight, and much less than with general anesthesia. You can see from the diagram that the spinal cord is separated from the epidural space by the dura (epidural means "above dura"), the subarachnoid space and the arachnoid. The dura and the arachnoid are both membranes that coat the length of the spinal cord from its base up to the brain. The anesthesiologist inserts the epidural needle very slowly and carefully so as not to puncture either of these membranes. If he or she punctures the first one, beyond the epidural space, the anesthesiologist will be able to feel the dura and also to see the appearance of liquid in the tube. This acts as a warning sign not to go any further. If the dura is punctured

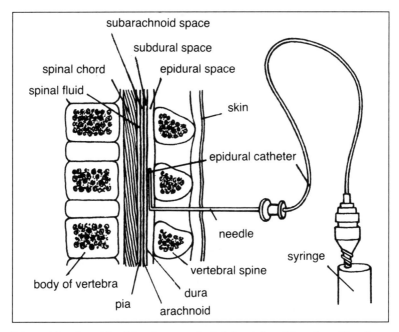

Figure 10. *An epidural involves anesthetic being injected into the epidural space in the spinal column. The epidural catheter is inserted through the skin of the back, between two vertebrae of the spine, into the epidural space. This cross-section of the spine shows that each vertebra is a hollow bone through which passes the spinal cord. The cord is protected by its spinal fluid and by 3 membranes, each of which has a space between it. The innermost is the pia, followed by the arachnoid, and lastly the dura, which is the membrane furthest from the spinal cord. An epidural effectively blocks the sensation of pain in the lower half of the body.*

in this way, no serious problems occur but the woman may develop a very painful headache which may persist for several days.

The dura is a thick outer protective coating for the spinal cord. Within this is the arachnoid, a very fine vascular membrane containing a lot of blood cells, which, if disturbed or punctured, will bleed (and cause headache). These two coatings cover the entire length of the spinal cord up into the brain. If either of them are disturbed, headache results. Headache after epidural is associated with a subdural tap (rather than epidural); in other words, the needle has gone beyond the dural space, through the dura. As a result, a small amount of blood may be lost from the membrane and find itself in the subarachnoid space. Alternatively, headache can be caused by a slight loss of spinal fluid from a subarachnoid puncture wound.

Once the tube (the epidural catheter) is threaded down the needle, you may feel a short, sharp pain, something like a minor electric shock, down one leg for a few seconds. This is caused by the catheter touching one of the nerves in the epidural space, but is nothing to worry about.

Once the epidural catheter is in place and the needle removed, local anesthetic can be introduced through it into the epidural space at intervals of an hour or two. These top-ups are best given by a trained specialist anesthesiologist, rather than someone unfamiliar with the technique. Top-ups are now sometimes replaced by an automatic infusion system, which is supervised by the anesthesiologist, giving a *continuous* small dose so that top-ups are no longer necessary.

Does it work?
Nearly 90% of women find that an epidural gives acceptable pain relief, but only some 50% find that pain is entirely relieved. The tube, the epidural catheter, being flexible, sometimes bends, and may therefore work only on one side of the body or not at all. The epidural sometimes fails because the catheter is in the wrong place, or the amount of anesthetic given is too little or is given too late.

The advantages of an epidural
An epidural may give complete relief from pain without loss of sensation, allowing you to remain fully conscious and involved with labor and delivery of your baby. It is safer for both mother and baby than a general anesthetic. It is particularly useful, therapeutically, for women who have incoordinate uterine action—in which contractions are ineffective and painful—thus prolonging the first stage of labor. An epidural, which can lower the blood pressure, is, incidentally, useful to women with high blood pressure and those who have pre-eclampsia. However, an epidural should not be given *in order to* lower the blood pressure in such cases. Severe pre-eclampsia can cause bleeding abnormalities and make an epidural unsafe, due to risks of bleeding into the epidural space.

The disadvantages of an epidural
An epidural should be given only by a skilled anesthesiologist (who should remain in attendance) and, ideally, only in the first stage of labor. It may fail, as in the case of a dural puncture. It may cause a sudden dip in blood pressure, although this should be identified by monitoring the mother's blood pressure and the baby's heartbeat, and the mother's blood pressure can then be treated.

Epidural anesthesia can also, occasionally, cause a number of other rare problems. If the subarachnoid space is entered, blood pressure may drop dramatically and the mother's heart stop, requiring immediate resuscitation. Very rarely, there is a severe allergic reaction to the anesthetic, or an overdose which may prove fatal. It is possible that the signs of a uterine rupture may not be obvious, particularly in a woman who has previously had a Cesarean, as an epidural would effectively mask the symptom of pain. Lastly, epidurals cannot be given to any woman who is, or could be hypovolemic (meaning a loss of circulating fluid), such as a woman who has lost a lot of blood or is very dehydrated. This is because the blood pressure may already be a bit low and the anesthetic will have a greater effect, thus possibly causing an even more reduced blood pressure; additionally, the anesthetic prevents the body responding and coping with hemorrhage.

However, even taking all these factors into account, an epidural is still much safer than a general anesthetic, particularly in the case of a complicated or Cesarean delivery. One hears of all sorts of alarming tales in connection with epidurals and the "medicalization" of birth, particularly from advocates of natural childbirth. One needs to put these tales in perspective, however, before one can make an informed decision about whether or not to have an epidural. It is only very rarely that something goes seriously wrong with an epidural. The situation is comparable to hearing of an aircrash. One hears about it only because it is out of the ordinary, an abnormal occurrence. Most people continue to take air flights because they know this.

There are several controversial issues surrounding the use of epidural anesthetics during labor. Some studies have suggested that epidurals may increase the risk of long labors, posterior presentations, and forceps deliveries. Other studies refute these points. However, most studies of epidurals do not account for the reason why the epidural was needed. For example, if epidurals are used for long painful labors (as opposed to short, fast labors), then obviously the conditions associated with long labors (including posterior presentations, tight fit through the pelvis, maternal exhaustion and poor pushing ability) will seem more common in women receiving epidurals.

Overall, most practitioners accustomed to working with epidurals do not feel they have consistent adverse effects on labor. However, they do acknowledge that many women do not "push" very effectively with epidurals in place. If a woman cannot push effectively, her attendant must either let the eipidural wear off, which prolongs labor, or help the baby out by vacuum extraction or forceps intervention. These procedures might have been avoided had the mother not had an epidural anesthetic.

In assessing the drawbacks or disadvantages of having an epidural, some women have mentioned a fear that paralysis or permanent injury could result. This has happened, but the chance of some serious consequence is very low indeed: In a survey of 500,000 epidurals, there was one case of permanent brain damage and one partial paralysis. In another survey of 27,000 epidurals, there were no such serious consequences. Both surveys showed that temporary urinary problems, backache, headache and temporary low blood pressure could occur. Low blood pressure is regarded as an ever-present hazard in epidural analgesia, while short-lived urinary problems, backache and headache occurred, in the larger survey, in 1 in 4,500 women. However, headache and backache can also occur in significant numbers after delivery under general anesthetic.

General anesthetic represents greater risks than an epidural or caudal, and this is why doctors now favor epidural anesthesia for operative vaginal deliveries and Cesarean deliveries, as well as for a number of other operations not related to midwifery.

COMPLEMENTARY TECHNIQUES

The chief complementary, nonmedical technique for the relief of pain is the control of breathing so that you breathe out over the height of the contraction, when pain may be at its most pronounced. In transcutaneous nerve stimulation (TNS), another complementary technique available in some hospitals, electrodes are held against your back and you operate a small machine, as and when you require it, to pass electrical current through the electrodes. The current is thought to stimulate the body's endorphins, the natural painkillers released within the body. Acupuncture and hypnosis may also work—it is certainly true that operations are carried out painlessly in China, using only acupuncture without any general anesthetic.

In the absence of scientific information to explain why acupuncture and hypnosis work, for example, some conventional doctors tend to feel that these methods are harmless—they don't have any side effects because they don't have *any* effect. An increasing number of doctors, however, are receptive to new ideas and feel that if the woman thinks they work, they do. So, if any of these things appeal to you, don't be intimidated by your doctor—go ahead and arrange with the hospital for the practitioner of your choice to be present for labor and delivery.

THE STAGES OF LABOR

Knowing when to go to the hospital, and recognizing the start of your labor, is discussed at the start of this chapter.

In the first stage of labor the cervix gradually dilates in response to the uterine contractions. The first stage of labor lasts between 6 and 12 hours if it is the first baby, and between 2 and 7 hours for a second or subsequent baby. It is best not to eat anything once labor has started just in case an anesthetic should later become necessary.

If, on the other hand, you have not recognized the first stage of labor, and you have eaten, and a general anesthetic does become necessary, you should tell the medical and nursing staff. They will *in any case* take the necessary safety procedures (which do *not* involve a stomach pump). This involves giving a drug, ranitidine, that inhibits acid secretion in the stomach. This means that if the contents of the stomach are regurgitated and the vomit inhaled, the vomit will be less in quantity and less acid in content, and therefore less injurious to the functioning of the lungs (it is the very powerful gastric acid that does the most damage).

You will find that contractions gradually become stronger and more painful. You may be able to cope with this by timing your breathing, as you have been taught, in accordance with each contraction. Towards the end of the first stage of labor, you may feel an urge to push, perhaps an overwhelming need to push, but it is then that you will be asked to pant or blow and refrain from pushing. This is when the midwife or doctor checks that the cervix is fully dilated.

In terms of technology, how much assistance you are given depends on your condition, the baby's condition and, to some extent, your wishes. Your blood pressure, temperature and pulse are checked by the nurse every 4 hours or so. An internal assessment will also be made to check the dilation of your cervix to make sure that labor is progressing. If no problems present themselves, you may only have on-off external fetal monitoring to check that the baby is all right. If there are difficulties or complications, you may have an intravenous drip (which conveys liquid by means of a tube fixed into a vein in your arm); frequent blood pressure measurements; continuous fetal monitoring, either external or internal; or delivery by forceps, which requires an episiotomy. The norm, however, is a vaginal, low- tech delivery, and this is what happens in 70% of all deliveries.

We have said that the amount of medical assistance you are given depends only partly upon your wishes. This is because, in cases of very difficult births, it may no longer be safe to realize the mother's wishes for a vaginal delivery, for example, or the avoidance of an episiotomy. If the only way to get the baby out is by forceps, this will be done before the baby is asphyxiated, and forceps delivery requires an episiotomy. If, as another example, it becomes clear that the baby cannot negotiate the birth canal and will die if it is left to struggle, an emergency Cesarean must be performed. At this point, the doctor should inform the mother of the decision and explain why the decision has been made.

So, once again, if anything is not clear to you, don't hesitate to ask, but do bear in mind that there are instances in which doctors have to take over in order to accomplish the successful delivery of a healthy baby. If they are compelled by the mother— who may not fully understand all the implications of the situation and who, in addition, may be distressed—to hold on, their scope for remedial action may be so compromised that the baby's or the mother's life is put in jeopardy.

The second stage of labor, in which the baby is born, is much shorter than the first. It usually lasts for anything up to 2 hours, and it is often much shorter. After you feel the first really expulsive contraction, at the end of the first stage of labor when you are asked not to push for a minute or two, you will then feel very powerful contractions, heralding the arrival of the baby. At this point, the technology for fetal monitoring and pain relief will be almost behind you, while matters including forceps (for about 15% of women) and episiotomy (for the majority) may be more immediate. The third stage of labor, described later in this chapter, usually follows quite quickly.

EPISIOTOMY

This surgical incision, or cut, is made into the perineum (the area between the vagina and the anus, and which includes some of the underlying structures of muscle and tissue) towards the end of the second stage of labor before the baby is born.

The cut is made primarily to relieve pressure on the muscle of the perineum (the perineal muscle, known as the levator muscle). It may be done straight down toward the rectum (midline) or in the lateral position (to one side) in order to avoid damage to the anal sphincter, which must remain intact in order to prevent the possibility of later incontinence of feces.

It is well known that spontaneous jagged tears can damage the levator muscle. This muscle is responsible for the control of bladder movements. It's the muscle you use to squeeze the last drop of urine out when you go to the toilet. You also use this muscle to contain yourself when you need to urinate but cannot do so immediately. If the muscle is permanently damaged, this control may be reduced or lost, with urinary incontinence the result.

The anal sphincter muscle is equally important as, if damaged, it can result in fecal incontinence, since it is no longer able to close. Waste matter then simply descends without being halted by the muscle.

An episiotomy is also made in order to prevent a subsequent prolapse, in which the muscles of the perineum, having been severely overstretched or torn, simply give up and the vagina then drops down protruding outside the body. An episiotomy may also be made because of the necessity for a forceps delivery, because the forceps would otherwise overstretch the muscles of the perineum and consequently damage them. It may also be made to reduce prolonged pressure of a rigid perineum on the baby's head in the second stage of labor.

For a midline episiotomy, a cut is made straight from the back of the vagina towards the rectum. Midline episiotomies heal quickly and are less painful than mediolateral ones. However, in the case of a woman with a short perineum or a very large baby, there is more risk of the episiotomy tearing into the rectum.

For a *mediolateral* episiotomy, the cut is made to the side (lateral position) in order to make sure that any deep tearing occurs laterally rather than longitudinally, and thus prevents damage to the anal sphincter muscle. A lateral cut is therefore made at 45° to the midline. This prevents the longitudinal, and jagged, tear that could occur if the cut were not made. It also ensures that any *subsequent* tearing, beyond the cut, at the point of birth of the baby's head, occurs laterally. In short, midline episiotomies heal more quickly and are less painful but allow less extra room than mediolateral episiotomies, and midline incisions carry a greater risk of rectal injury. It is reasonable to ask your doctor which he or she prefers and why. (See Figure 11.)

Episiotomy is not done solely for the convenience of doctors, although it is of course easier to repair a straight cut than a tear, and thus more likely to be accurately done. If an uncontrolled tear occurs, it may occur both to left and right of the vagina, and the vulva and labia may also be badly torn. Sewing up this kind of tear is like trying to put a jigsaw back together and requires considerable skill and experience. Episiotomy is done, therefore, to eliminate the need for this, and as a precaution with preventative medicine in mind. A summary of the main reasons follows:

1. in order to prevent tearing of underlying muscle, i.e. in order to prevent possible prolapse or incontinence (as explained above);
2. when the baby's head becomes stuck on the perineum and can move no further;
3. fetal distress, when the baby must be born immediately;
4. an impending perineal tear, when it can be seen that the perineum is stretched to the limit but the baby's head has still not appeared;
5. forceps or vacuum extraction (ventouse) delivery (discussed later in this chapter);
6. breech presentation;
7. in women who have had, in a previous pregnancy, a severe tear or extensive perineal repair;
8. in women with raised blood pressure or a heart condition, in order to shorten labor;
9. maternal exhaustion, in which the mother is worn out and dispirited and, therefore, no longer able to push.

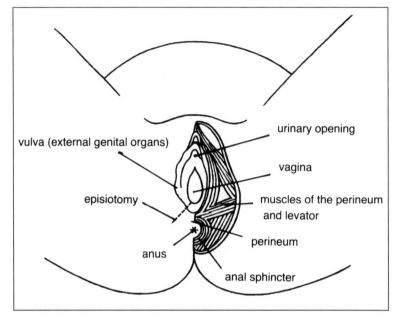

Figure 11. *The dotted line shows where the cut for an episiotomy is normally made. An episiotomy is intended to prevent the surrounding muscles being torn in order that incontinence and prolapse in later life can be avoided, and to prevent undue delay in the birth of the baby.*

How an episiotomy is performed

The area of the vagina and anus is injected with local anesthetic, unless an epidural is already in place. A cut is made at the onset of a contraction as the baby's head advances on the perineum. The incision starts in the midline and then passes backwards and laterally to avoid incising the anal sphincter or straight down if there is enough room.

The baby's head appears, you are told not to push, the cord is checked and the baby's head helped out. After the baby is born, your anal area is injected with more local anesthetic and the various layers of skin and muscle are drawn together exactly, it is to be hoped, as they were before and neatly stitched. It is true that some bleeding, bruising and, occasionally, infection may result from an episiotomy.

Avoiding an episiotomy

Whether or not an episiotomy can be avoided rather depends on why it is being proposed. For example, if you are told: "Well, it's simply routine," you may elect, if you wish, not to have one. If, on the other hand, it is to be performed for one of the reasons listed above (on page 149), it may be unavoidable. If the baby's head is stuck on the perineum, for example, there are only minutes in which to free it and deliver it, and the woman who refuses an episiotomy in this situation risks losing her baby.

The most important thing you can do, which may help to avoid an episiotomy, is to do regular pelvic floor muscles and the other exercises specifically useful in pregnancy, as described in Chapter 3. This helps to ensure that all your muscles, including those of the perineum, are of good tone and therefore capable of being stretched to the limit without tearing.

It may also be that preparing for birth in the squatting position helps to prevent the need for an episiotomy. Squatting promotes the relaxation of the pelvic floor and an improved blood flow, which means that the contractions are more effective, which means, in turn, that both forceps and episiotomy may be avoided. In the squatting position, the law of gravity assists the descent of the baby's presenting part which, in this position, exerts the maximum pressure upon the cervix. With all this in mind, women with low-risk pregnancies who are having on-off external fetal monitoring, may well benefit by being free to move about and to adopt a squatting position if they wish to do so.

THE BIRTH

When you are told *not* to push, you will know that you are at last very close to seeing your baby. Once the cord has been checked, and the baby's head helped out—when you can put your hand down and touch the baby for the first time— the rest of the birth follows quickly with less discomfort. The baby may cry immediately—a good sign—and its mouth and nose will be cleared of mucus and fluid by the midwife or doctor, the cord will be clamped and cut, and the baby handed to you, so that you see and hold her or him within a minute or two of the birth.

THE THIRD STAGE OF LABOR

The placenta is delivered in the final stage of labor with another contraction. You may be given an injection of Syntocinon and/or an ergot derivative to make the uterus contract, in order to prevent post-partum hemorrhage; if the uterus does not contract, hemorrhage after the birth can occur, particular so in twin or multiple births when the uterus may have been stretched to the limit. The birth attendant sometimes assists delivery of the placenta by gently pulling on the umbilical cord, by depressing your abdominal area and by asking you to push—just one more time. (It is at this point that you will be stitched, if necessary, as explained above, under the heading of *Episiotomy*.) Occasionally, the placenta does not detach from the wall of the uterus and may have to be removed manually under general anesthetic, or with an epidural.

COMPLICATIONS

The majority of pregnancies result in the successful delivery of a healthy baby, but complications can sometimes arise. If these are of a nature that can be anticipated before labor starts, you may have an assisted vaginal delivery or a Cesarean delivery, as described in the previous chapter. Other complications may not be apparent, however, until labor is well under way. These include prolonged labor, leading to fetal distress, maternal distress or both; a slow or dysfunctional labor in which nothing much happens; a labor with short, sharp contractions and severe backache (possibly caused by the baby assuming a posterior position); the baby's head not well flexed or in an unusual position; a rigid pelvis or some other abnormality; or a prolapsed cord, when the cord is below the baby's head.

Any of these complications may require medical assistance in the form of emergency Cesarean delivery, forceps delivery and/or episiotomy. An emergency Cesarean is essentially the same operation as described in the previous chapter, but carried out without advance planning in an atmosphere, consequently, of greater anxiety for the mother. Episiotomy, and the reasons for it, have been described earlier in this chapter. This brings us to forceps delivery, and its more unusual alternative, vacuum extraction (also known as ventouse delivery).

FORCEPS DELIVERY

A pair of forceps looks somewhat like a pair of tongs or a pair of spoons. If there is a delay in the second stage of labor, they are passed up through the vagina and gently applied either side of the baby's head so that the baby can be drawn gently and slowly down the birth canal and delivered without delay. Difficulties besetting normal vaginal delivery can often be anticipated these days, so that fewer forceps and more Cesarean deliveries are performed. Forceps tend to be used only in those borderline cases in which vaginal delivery was expected and in which, in light of labor, it can be seen that the baby needs some assistance, but in which it is anticipated that a Cesarean can still be avoided.

A forceps delivery takes from 2 to 10 minutes, depending upon the degree of difficulty and, to some extent, on the skill of the obstetrician. It is not usually difficult but it does require skill and should therefore be performed only by experienced obstetricians. A fully prepared operating room should be available if the technique fails. In such cases, minutes can be crucial.

The majority of forceps deliveries are reasonably easy and should be attempted only if the baby's head is already in the pelvis. If the baby's head is already quite low down, it takes only a couple of minutes to make an episiotomy, apply the forceps and deliver the baby. It happens so quickly that the mother is scarcely aware of what is happening until after the event.

At the second level of difficulty, when the baby's head may still be higher in the pelvis, a pudendal block will be given (see *Relief from pain* earlier in this chapter), or an epidural (if the instruments are already set up), or possibly, in the last resort, a general anesthetic, in cases in which it is not known whether the forceps technique will succeed. This is known as a "trial of forceps" and is carried out with a fully prepared operating room available should it be needed.

At the third level of difficulty, if the baby's head is in an awkward position (such as occipito-posterior or transverse), it must rotate in order to allow vaginal delivery. The baby cannot be born vaginally otherwise. It is sometimes possible to rotate the baby's head manually or with forceps. If it is not clear whether this is going to succeed, a trial of forceps may be carried out, with general or epidural anesthetic, and Cesarean the course of action adopted if it does not.

The two main reasons for performing a forceps delivery are when the second stage of labor has become prolonged and/or fetal distress in which the baby becomes progressively starved of oxygen. For example, the baby's head may start to descend and then become stuck on the perineum or, earlier, in the pelvic cavity. In such cases, it may be possible to avoid a Cesarean with the judicious use of forceps. However, the forceps necessarily distend the vagina and the perineum and it is therefore good, and normal, medical practice to make an episiotomy first.

VACUUM EXTRACTION (VENTOUSE)

This method of last-minute medical assistance, when the baby is in difficulties or the mother exhausted, involves a small cup being passed up the vagina and attached by suction to the baby's head, suction being induced by means of a small hand pump. The cup is then pulled gently, usually resulting in the birth of the baby. You would have a local anesthetic first, but there is no need for an episiotomy, unless the reason for the delayed birth of the baby itself necessitates it. This procedure requires a certain amount of skill, particularly in the application of the cup. If the vacuum extraction technique does not work, it should be abandoned after 20 minutes.

Vacuum extraction is sometimes preferred to forceps because it is kinder to the tissues of the vagina and cervix. It is also safer than a Cesarean. A chignon-shaped swelling may be apparent on the baby's head for a while after delivery, but this is not serious and will subside. More serious damage can, very rarely, occur to the baby with the use of this instrument, so vacuum extraction will usually be carried out only by someone experienced in its use.

ACHIEVED IT AT LAST!

There is a very good chance that you will have a straightforward labor and delivery, and you should perhaps not worry too much about complications that could occur but are much more likely not to. You will probably feel an overwhelming sense of relief, elation and fatigue, when at last your baby is given to you to hold.

You will probably be left alone with your partner and the baby for a while—hospital practice varies in this and it will depend partly on how you and the baby are. At some point, your pulse and blood pressure will be checked and your temperature will be taken. The baby will be weighed and measured and given a name band shortly after delivery, and he or she will be assessed according to the Apgar score, shown below.

HOW'S THE BABY?

After delivery the first priority is to make sure that the baby is breathing. It is then weighed and measured and at some point assessed according to the Apgar score. Five things are checked, as an indication of the baby's general health, and points awarded from 0 to 2 for each of the 5 factors. The baby that scores 7 or above is in good general health. The 5 signs are: respiratory effort (breathing); pulse rate; color (pallor); muscular tone; and response to stimuli (reflexes). Testing according to this score may be repeated after 5 minutes.

Table 11.3

Sign	0	1	2
Respiratory effort	none	weak cry, slow breathing	good strong cry
Pulse (heart rate)	none	slow, under 100 beats per minute	fast (over 100 per minute)
Color (pallor)	blue-pale	good body color with blue fingers and toes	good color, including pink fingers and toes
Muscular tone	limp	some flexing of fingers and toes	active, fingers and toes flexing well
Response to stimuli (reflex irritability)	no response	grimace	cry

Newborn babies often don't look completely beautiful except perhaps to their parents, until a few days after their birth when the minor bumps and wrinkles, caused by the journey down the birth canal, have smoothed out. So don't be surprised if your baby has little bruises, the odd spot or rash and, possibly, enlarged breasts and genitals (caused by hormonal fluctuations which settle soon after birth). The umbilical cord will be clamped and cut and the clamped stump at the baby's navel left to drop off of its own accord.

If breast-feeding works for you and your baby, this will be encouraged in the hospital. If you experience any problems (see Chapter 8), don't hesitate to ask for guidance and support—the technique does not always come naturally.

Before you leave the hospital, the baby will be given a test for phenylketonuria. This is a disease which, if untreated, causes a child to be mentally impaired. The disease is simply detected by taking a small blood sample from the baby and analyzing it. If the disease is found to be present, the baby can be treated with complete success.

If the mother has tuberculosis, or is likely to have been exposed to TB, the baby will be offered a BCG vaccination shortly after delivery. The babies of women with hepatitis B will be given hepatitis B vaccine and an immune globulin injection.

WHAT HAPPENS NOW?

Women that need special care, such as diabetics and those with raised blood pressure, may stay in the hospital a little longer than others, until they are well enough to leave. A rhesus-negative woman who has delivered a rhesus-positive baby will be given an Rh immune globulin injection to destroy any antibodies that may have appeared in her blood, as these would threaten a subsequent pregnancy. If the mother is not immune to rubella, she will now be given a rubella injection and warned not to become pregnant for three months.

The length of time that a woman stays in the hospital these days varies greatly from 6 hours after delivery (if it is the second or subsequent child, and if there are no problems) to 2 or 3 days if it is a first child, and perhaps up to 10 in some cases.

HOW DO YOU FEEL?

Some women feel nothing but elation and satisfaction at the birth of their babies, but many feel anything but elated. Baby blues, when you feel weepy for no reason obvious to you, together with a sense of helplessness, are so common that the condition is regarded as normal. However, if you do feel awful, do confide in someone—a nurse, a doctor, your partner or whoever you feel is most approachable. Above all, don't hesitate while you are in the hospital to ask questions about feeding, any pains you may have; and ask for treatment, if necessary, for constipation, hemorrhoids or anything else that is bothering you.

GOING HOME

You may be delighted to relax in your normal environment once again, but at the same time it is possible, particularly if it is your first baby, that the newness and the responsibility of your changed situation combine to make you feel a little overwhelmed at times. This is caused partly by the action of your hormones, as they settle down once again to their normal levels and partly because everything *is* new to you. The baby has but two thoughts on its mind at this time—breast and bowel—and you may feel that this is a demanding time, when the baby needs regular feeding every few hours and her or his diapers changed regularly, with bouts of bellyache, boredom and crying in between. This acute stage does not usually last for more than about 3 months, but that can seem like a long time.

Do talk to your friends and family, or your doctor if anything bothers you or if you feel a bit down. Meanwhile, don't neglect your own diet and your own health, while you are concentrating upon your baby. Look back to Chapter 3 and think about eating for health (and energy), exercise and fresh air, and relaxation, so that you, and your partner, may enjoy your baby to the fullest.

Appendix: Genetic Disorders

The five main methods of prenatal diagnosis for genetic disorders are amniocentesis; fetoscopy; alphafetoprotein level measurement; chorionic villus sampling; and detailed ultrasound scan. The first three methods are discussed in Chapter 7, while the remaining two are described in Chapter 5.

These tests can be used to identify a very large number of genetic disorders, as shown below. It must be emphasized that the majority of these disorders is rare and, in many cases, women are tested only if their family medical history suggests it or if a routine test at the prenatal clinic merits further investigation.

Chromosomal
Down's syndrome, trisomies 13 and 18, and other autosomal trisomies
Klinefelter's syndrome and other sex chromosome aneuploidy in males
Turner's syndrome, XXX syndrome, and other sex chromosome aneuploidy in females
Chromosome deletions or rearrangements, balanced or aneuploid
Fragile (X) syndrome

Congenital malformation
Neural tube defect and severe microcephaly or hydrocephaly
Cardiac defect

Renal agenesis, cystic kidney, hydronephrosis, prune belly, *exstrophy of the bladder
Tracheo-oesophageal stenosis and fistula, exomphalos and gastro-schisis, diaphragmatic hernia, duodenal atresia
Skeletal dysplasia
Cleft lip or palate
Cystic hygroma, teratomas, and fetal hydrops
Numerous multiple congenital anomaly syndromes

Single gene defects with known gene product
Sickle cell disease and thalassemias

Inborn errors of metabolism
Mucopolysaccharidoses

Aminoacidopathies:
  Phenylketonuria
  Ornithine carbamyl tranferase
    deficiency
  Citrullinuria
  Argininosuccinicaciduria
  Homocystinuria
  Maple syrup urine disease
Carbohydrate disorders:
  Galactosemia
  Galactokinase and galactose 4-
    epimerase deficiency
  Glycogenoses
Purine and pyrimidine disorders:
  Lesch-Nyhan syndrome
  Adenine phosphoribosyl trans-
    ferase deficiency
Organic acidurias:
  Methylmalonic acidurias
  Proprionic acidemia
  3-Methylcrotonyl coenzyme A
    carboxylase deficiency
Lipid disorders:
  Anderson-Fabry disease
  Farber's disease
  Fucosidosis
  Gangliosidoses
  Gaucher's disease
  I cell disease
  Krabbe's disease
  Mannosidosis
  Metachromatic leucodystrophy
  Mucolipidosis III
  Niemann-Pick disease
  Sialidosis
  Wolman's disease
Other
  Acid phosphatasia
  Adrenal hyperplasia (21-
    hydroxylase deficiency)
  Cerebrohepatorenal syn drome
  Cystinosis
Hypophosphatasia
Placental steroid sulphatase defi-
  ciency (X linked ichthyosis)

Coagulation defects
Hemophilia A and B
Factor X deficiency

Immune deficiency disorders
Severe combined immunodefi-
  ciency syndrome
T cell immunodeficiency

Collagen disorders
Ehlers-Danlos syndrome types II
  and V (some cases)

**Single gene defects with
  unknown gene product**
Cystic fibrosis
Duchenne and Becker types of
  dystrophy
Huntington's chorea
Adult polycystic kidney
  disease
Generalized neurofibromatosis
  (von Recklinghausen's
  disease)
Myotonic dystrophy
Ataxia telangiectasia
Bloom's syndrome
Fanconi's anemia
Robert's syndrome
Xeroderma pigmentosum
Epidermolysis bullosa
  syndromes
Hypohidrotic ectodermal
  dysplasia
Congenital nephrosis (Finnish
  type)
Multiple endocrine neoplasias

Fetal infections
Intrauterine rubella
Intrauterine cytomegalovirus

Other
a1 Antitrypsin deficiency
Acute intermittent porphyria

*Lower urinary tract obstruction with a greatly enlarged bladder distend-
ing the abdomen.

Reproduced by kind permission of Dr. M. d'A Crawfurd and the *British Medical Journal.*

Further Reading

This small and selective choice of books may be of interest to those women who are pregnant or intend to be so.

Eisenberg, Arlene, Murkoff, Heidi Eisenberg and Hathaway, Sandee Eisenberg. *What to Expect When You're Expecting.* New York: Workman, 1988.

Grams, Marilyn. *Breastfeeding Source Book: Where to Get What You Need to Breastfeed Successfully.* Sheridan, WY: Achievement Press, 1988.

Harrison, Helen and Kositsky, Ann. *The Premature Baby Book.* New York: St. Martin's, 1983.

Junor, Penny. *What Every Woman Needs to Know: Facts and Fears About Pregnancy, Childbirth and Womanhood.* North Pomfret, Vermont: David & Charles, 1989.

La Leche League International. *The Womanly Art of Breastfeeding.* Franklin Park, Illinois: La Leche League International, 1987.

Lauwers, Judith. *Breastfeeding Today: A Mother's Companion.* Wayne, New Jersey: Avery, 1987.

Leach, Penelope. *Your Baby and Child.* Rev. New York: Knopf, 1989.

Ting, Rosalind. *The Complete Mothercare Manual: An Illustrated Guide to Pregnancy, Birth & Childcare.* Englewood Cliffs, New Jersey: Prentice-Hall, 1987.

INDEX